Statistics in Small Doses

D1392336

For Churchill Livingstone:

Commissioning Editor: Michael Parkinson
Project Editor: Janice Urquhart
Copy Editor: Michael Fitch
Project Controller: Kay Hunston
Design Direction: Erik Bigland
Sales Promotion Executive: Marion Pollock

Statistics in Small Doses

Win M. Castle

MD FFPP MB BS MIS MFCM
(Retired) Vice President of International
Drug Surveillance, Glaxo Research Institute,
Research Triangle Park, North Carolina, USA

Philip M. North

BSc MSc PhD CStat
Managing Director

ASRU LTD

APPLIED STATISTICS RESEARCH UNIT

University of Kent at Canterbury, England, UK

THIRD EDITION

CHURCHILL LIVINGSTONE
EDINBURGH HONG KONG LONDON MADRID MELBOURNE NEW YORK AND
TOKYO 1995

CHURCHILL LIVINGSTONE
Medical Division of Pearson Professional Limited

Distributed in the United States of America by
Churchill Livingstone Inc., 650 Avenue of the
Americas, New York, N. Y. 10011, and by associated
companies, branches and representatives
throughout the world.

© Pearson Professional Limited 1995

First published 1995

ISBN 0 443 04542 9

British Library Cataloguing in Publication Data
A catalogue record for this book is available from the
British Library

Library of Congress Cataloging in Publication Data
A catalog record for this book is available from the
Library of Congress

The
publisher's
policy is to use
**paper manufactured
from sustainable forests**

Produced by Longman Singapore Publishers (Pte) Ltd.
Printed in Singapore.

Contents

Preface

Many medical and pharmaceutical workers – be they staff or research students – do not have, through no fault of their own, a good knowledge of statistics. Yet their subject is such that statistics is one of the tools most commonly used in it. So those workers need to have, at the very least, a good understanding of what statistics is all about and of what procedures will be used under what circumstances. Often they will find themselves reading about statistical tests and results in the medical literature, so they need to know what they are reading about and to have a critical eye when seeing results presented. The aim of this book is to address those needs for such people. The examples in the book have a medical bias, to set an appropriate context for medical workers, but they can be easily understood by non-medical people as well, and the book should also be of benefit to such people. This is the third edition of a book first published over twenty years ago and the book has been much used over that time. For this edition the text has been thoroughly revised and updated.

The book is intended for those who wish to make a start along statistical paths, and is likely to be especially relevant to those wishing to do so in a medical context. We have purposely chosen to use numerical examples which are an over-simplification of reality to clarify the points being made in the text. We have wanted to ensure that it is simple, through use of the numerical examples, to understand the principles involved, rather than run the risk of the unfamiliar reader becoming confused by mathematical gymnastics when he/she is still unclear about the basic ideas of the subject.

We have covered those topics which seem to be most useful to medical workers. New topics have been added, compared with the earlier editions, where this seemed appropriate and necessary.

The first part of the book should be easy going for all readers. This is deliberate, because just as an examination candidate is reassured by being able to answer the first few questions in the paper, so are readers of a book reassured by being able to understand the first few chapters, when the book is about a subject which they perceive – rightly or wrongly – to be difficult. Practical examples are included, to enable readers to test their skills without the prompts included in the text.

This book is presented in the main in the form of a programmed learning text. The information is dispensed in small doses called 'frames' and this is done by means of questions and answers designed to test continuously the reader's grasp of the subject matter. In order to derive maximum benefit the reader is advised to attempt to answer the questions in each frame before looking at the given responses. This can be easily arranged since the answers are all listed in the shaded section on the right-hand side of each page – so these sections can be covered up with a piece of paper or card. Where it has been felt to be helpful to add further explanation or comments, to give a more complete background to the points being made, these have been included with the answers. Some particularly important points have been emphasised in the book by repeatedly asking questions about them, to the extent that they should become thoroughly familiar to the reader, who should then easily retain the information in his/her memory, ready for immediate recall.

Because the book is presented as a programmed learning text, an index is not provided, since the intention is that the reader should study the book as a whole, rather than dipping into parts of it. One point leads on to the next in the text in a quite deliberate fashion, the reader continuously building on information already assimilated from earlier frames. However, at the end of each chapter is a revision summary which fully indicates the contents of that particular chapter.

Chapters 19 (on simple linear regression), 21 (on nonparametric methods) and 22 (on statistical computing) in this edition are new. The form of presentation in Chapter 19 especially is intended to prepare those readers who wish to go on to read somewhat more advanced texts on the subject for what they are likely to meet. Development of the material in that chapter is through the concept of a statistical model, which is so important in statistical methods which follow on from the contents of this book.

The original book was developed over a period of four years and its first published form was its 7th amended version. The contents of the original teaching frames were thoroughly validated in practical use, so it has not seemed sensible to change them greatly in the present edition, though emphasis has been changed in some places, where appropriate. Criticism and advice were received and taken into account at every stage and we should like to thank all those who read the text so conscientiously during its development. To a large extent, these people have written the book. We thank them and at the same time exonerate them from any blame for errors, which are our own responsibility. Early comments were received from medical students and colleagues of WMC at the Royal Free Hospital Medical School and at the Universities of Leeds, Pretoria and Witwatersrand. In the University of Zimbabwe, besides considerable assistance from within the Faculty of Medicine, groups of undergraduates and graduates in the Faculties of Science and Education studied and commented on the early versions. For this latest edition we are indebted to Dr Alexa Laurence of ASRU Ltd at the University of Kent for reviewing the whole text, and concentrating especially on the new sections, and to Owen Roberts, also of ASRU Ltd, for assistance with the diagrams. Thanks are also due to Debbie Kent, again of ASRU Ltd, for her seemingly endless patience and good nature when typing the new edition.

Any errors that remain after all this are the responsibility of the authors.

P. M. N.
1995

1. Types of results: counts and measurements

INTRODUCTION

Welcome to this programmed learning text. Make sure that you work through frame by frame in sequence and try to answer the questions in the frames. The answers in the shaded frames should be covered up initially, to test your ability to answer the questions yourself.

This chapter teaches you to distinguish between the two main types of numerical data – counts and measurements – as this distinction is used over and over again throughout this book. Rates, ratios, proportions and percentages are also described briefly.

1.1	The height of a patient is *measured*. The number of patients attending a particular clinic is *counted*.	
	Is weight measured or counted?	Measured
	What about time of survival?	Measured
	Are people who have been vaccinated usually measured or counted?	Counted

1.2	Results which are measured are called *quantitative*. When each individual has one measurement ascribed to him/her from a continuous spectrum, e.g. heights of 1.50 m, 1.70 m, 1.88 m, the data are also called *continuous*. Results which allot people or any other subjects into groups with certain attributes are called *qualitative*. Any kinds of data in the form of counts are called *discrete*.	

1.3	What kind of data is sex?	Qualitative and discrete (in that an individual is included either with males or females).
	What kind of data is the number of decayed teeth in a person's mouth?	Discrete (because it is a count).
	What kind of result is heart size?	Quantitative and continuous (because it is measured).

1.4	What kind of result is red cell volume?	Quantitative
1.5	Why is it quantitative?	Because it is measured.
1.6	Blood groups are................data.	Qualitative, since patients are allotted into particular groups.
1.7	Write down 3 different sources of quantitative measurement, e.g. bladder capacity. (1) .... (2) .... (3)	Systolic blood pressure, body temperature and weight are 3 possibilities. There are many others.
1.8	Sometimes examination results are listed qualitatively rather than quantitatively. How is this done?	Candidates are grouped on a pass/fail basis only, or are put into grades.

1.9   Country of origin and sex of doctors practising in a newly developed African country.

Country of origin	Sex		
	Male	Female	Total
England & Wales	142	28	170
Ireland	29	2	31
Italy	5	3	8
Scotland	74	15	89
S. Africa	157	26	183
U.S.A.	5	1	6
Others	7	10	17
Total	419	85	504

What type of data are these?   Qualitative

We say that the doctors are *classified* in two different ways, i.e. by country of origin and by sex. The table depicting such a cross-classification is called a *contingency table*.

1.10	From the table, how many doctors originated in England and Wales?	170

1.11	Qualitative results are sometimes expressed as a ratio, a proportion or a percentage. Any group we single out for mention can be said to have the 'characteristic mentioned' (e.g. doctors originating in England and Wales). If we call this group the sheep, for illustration, we might think of the others as the goats. Which are the goats in the last frame?	Doctors in the African country originating outside England and Wales.

1.12   A *ratio* takes the following form:

$$\frac{\text{the number of sheep}}{\text{the number of goats}},$$

often expressed as the number of sheep : the number of goats.
Using the 'sheep' and 'goats' labelling that we used in the above table, what does this ratio become there?

$\frac{170}{334} = \frac{85}{167}$, which may be expressed as
85 : 167
or 85 to 167

In Frame 1.9 what is the ratio of those who originated in England and Wales to those who did not?

$\frac{170}{334} = \frac{85}{167}$, or 85 : 167 (85 to 167), as above.

1.13   What is the ratio of women to men doctors in the African country?

$\frac{85}{419}$, or 85 : 419 (85 to 419)

1.14   If $\dfrac{\text{the number of sheep}}{\text{the number of goats}}$ is a ratio,

and $\dfrac{\text{the number of sheep}}{\text{the number of sheep and goats}}$ is a proportion,

then
$\dfrac{\text{the red cell volume}}{\text{the total blood volume}}$ is a ....

proportion
Note that

$\dfrac{\text{the red cell volume}}{\text{the white cell volume}}$
is a ratio.

1.14 *cont'd*
Note that what is being done in the proportion is comparing the number of subjects with a particular attribute with the total number of subjects.

1.15 The ratio of women doctors to men in the African country

is $\dfrac{85}{419}$ or 85 : 419.

What is the proportion?

$$\frac{85}{419 + 85} = \frac{85}{504}$$
This may be expressed as 0.17.

1.16 $100 \times \dfrac{183}{504}$

is the percentage (%) of all doctors in the African country who originated in South Africa. The percentage is defined as 100 times the ....

proportion

1.17 In our illustrative terminology, is the percentage therefore

$100 \times \dfrac{\text{the number of sheep}}{\text{the number of goats}}$?

No. The percentage is

$100 \times \dfrac{\text{the number of sheep}}{\text{the number of sheep and goats}}$.

1.18 Give names to the following indices from Frame 1.9. (They all refer to the U.S.A.)

(a) $\dfrac{1}{85}$ (b) $\dfrac{1}{84}$ (c) $\dfrac{100}{85}$

The (a) proportion, (b) ratio and (c) percentage of women doctors in the African country who originated in the U.S.A.

1.19 It is perfectly in order to cancel the numerator and denominator where possible.

$\dfrac{100}{85}$% can be written ....

$1\dfrac{3}{17}$% or 1.2%

1.20 Ratios, proportions and percentages may seem innocent. They are sometimes misused in journals. For example, an ear, nose and throat

Not until you know how many patients are involved. He may have only operated once!

1.20   *cont'd*
surgeon proudly reports that he has a 100% 5-year survival rate for patients with cancer of the throat after operation. Are you impressed?

Unless the actual number involved is also quoted mistrust ratios, proportions and percentages.

1.21   A normal blood picture should contain about 5 million red cells and 5 thousand white ones, i.e. a ratio of

$$\frac{1000}{1}, \text{ or } 1000 : 1.$$

Mr Van der Werwe's blood cells are in the ratio 1000 to 1. Should we infer that his blood picture is satisfactory?

You cannot say. He may have 5 million white cells and leukaemia if the direction of the ratio is not specified. A ratio on its own is not enough.

1.22   Besides ratios, proportions and percentages, doctors quote 'rates'. For example, the still-birth rate is

$$\frac{\text{the number of still-births}}{\text{the total number of births}} \times 1000$$

Is this a percentage, a proportion or a ratio?

None of these. It is 10 times the percentage. It is the number of events of interest per thousand of the 'population' concerned – in this case, the number of still-births per thousand births.

1.23   Some of the so-called 'rates' in Medicine are not true rates, a rate being defined as

$$\frac{\text{the number counted over a certain period}}{\text{the total at a given time}}$$

The crude death rate is calculated from

$$\frac{\text{the number of deaths in a year}}{\text{the estimated population on July 1st}}$$

Is this a proper rate?

Yes. (The given definition is usually multiplied by 1000.)

1.24 $\dfrac{\text{The number of deaths by accident in 1066}}{\text{The number of survivors in 1066}}$

is a rate/ratio/proportion?   ratio

1.25   Ratios, rates, proportions and   Qualitative
       percentages are all means of expressing
       what kind of data?

1.26   If you are presented with any of these   The number involved in
       values what should you also be told?   the survey or trial

1.27   Occasionally in medical journals the
       terms ratio, proportion and rate are
       confused. One may read that the ratio of
       A to B is 10% instead of one to ....   nine

$$\frac{A}{A + B} \times 100 = 10\%$$

$$\therefore \frac{A}{A + B} = \frac{1}{10}$$

$$\therefore 10A = A + B$$

$$\therefore 9A = B$$

$$\therefore \frac{A}{B} = \frac{1}{9}$$

1.28   A expressed as a proportion is defined as   Total, say $A + B$
       $\dfrac{A}{?}$

1.29   If A expressed as a proportion *increases*
       and this is

       $\dfrac{A}{A + B}$, then B expressed as a proportion

       must increase/decrease at the same   decrease
       time?

1.30   One of us read in a journal: It is inevitable rather than
       'It is particularly interesting to see that as   interesting. Like a salary
       the proportion of live eggs increases the   cheque, as the proportion
       proportion of dead eggs decreases.'   of tax increases the
       Comment.   proportion of spending

<table>
<tr><td>1.30</td><td>cont'd</td><td>money must decrease. Keep your eyes open in case you spot this type of mistake in the journals, though it is less likely now than it was some years ago as the statistical refereeing of such papers is now more stringent.</td></tr>
</table>

1.31   Before learning about how to present qualitative results (and how not to!) in the next chapter, check that you have learnt all the main points in this chapter in the Revision Summary below.

SUMMARY

Results which are counted into groups are qualitative. Quantitative values are measured. The difference is important from the statistical point of view – they are illustrated as well as being analysed differently.

Qualitative data can be summarised as

ratios, of the form $\dfrac{sheep}{goats}$, and proportions, of the form $\dfrac{sheep}{total}$, or

percentages, where the percentage (%) is 100 times the proportion.

It is wrong to state one of these indices without quoting the number of subjects involved. A rate is similar to a proportion but its denominator is a static measurement whereas the numerator is counted over a period of time. In fact in medical practice the two most commonly used morbidity rates, the prevalence and the incidence, are often confused. Basically the *prevalence* rate tells us how common is a situation whereas the *incidence* tells us how often the situation occurs. As an example of the difference between the terms, consider the pregnancy rate in a community of rabbits in a given year, 1993. The incidence of pregnancy is the number of rabbits becoming pregnant during 1993 divided by the number of rabbits exposed to risk during that year. The prevalence has the same denominator but the numerator is all those rabbits that are pregnant during 1993 – unlike the incidence it includes those rabbits becoming pregnant during 1992 that delivered their offspring in 1993. Prevalence rates themselves can be pinpointed to answer the question how common is the situation at a particular moment in time – the 'point' prevalence as opposed to the 'period' prevalence which includes all those in the given situation over a period of time.

2. Illustrating counts

INTRODUCTION

Sometimes research workers spend a lot of their time obtaining results but then present them poorly. Illustrating data is a useful topic to consider here as badly presented results can mislead you. Diagrams should aid the reader by saving him/her time and by highlighting points. Qualitative and quantitative data are presented differently and in this chapter we learn about illustrating counts, then in the subsequent chapter, illustrating measurements. Inspection of diagrams of the data is very important for 'getting to know the data', as part of a more general exploratory data analysis, often referred to as EDA. It is particularly important to carry out this stage of the analysis, especially in an age where it is all too easy to run data through analyses in computer packages. The danger here is that the packages may be inappropriately used, and yet appear to produce credible results. Attention paid to looking at the data carefully and thoroughly will help to minimise such risks.

2.1 There are 4 common ways of presenting qualitative, i.e. counted, data. These are:

(a) Pie diagram
(b) Pictogram
(c) Bar chart
(d) Proportional bar chart

These 4 methods are used below to illustrate the fact that in a particular population:

45% have blood group O
41% have blood group A
10% have blood group B
 4% have blood group AB

Can you label the methods? (You will need to guess, using the list above.)

2.1   *cont'd*

(a) pie diagram
(b) proportional bar chart
(c) bar chart
(d) pictogram

If your answers are correct you may go straight to Frame 2.5.

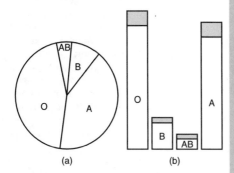

(a) is a .... (b) is a ....

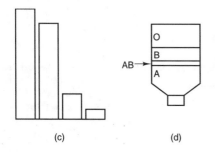

(c) is a .... (d) is a ....

2.2   Why is (a) called a pie diagram?

It is pie-shaped.

2.3   Why is (c) called a bar chart?

It is shaped like a series of bars.

2.4   Why is (b) called a proportional bar chart?

It is a bar chart with subdivisions proportioned off, corresponding to some subgroups of interest.

2.5   (d) is a pictogram. The 'gram' infers measurement and 'picto' a picture. What picture would you use to represent the composition of cows' milk by volume?

A milk bottle or an urn are possibilities. Alternatively you may choose to draw a cow, though this would be difficult to subdivide in a visually recognisable way. (Numbers of small cows might be used, however, to compare milk production in

2.5 *cont'd*

different EC countries, say.) Pictograms can be useful for making comparisons (e.g. to show how the total hospital budget is subdivided over various categories of spending, in two different hospitals). In the example quoted, the total *area* of each diagram may be made proportional to the total budget, *not* the linear dimensions, since this would lead to distortion (e.g. doubling the size of the linear dimensions increases the area fourfold). Note the possibilities for malpractice here!

2.6 What method of representation is this?

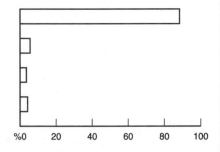

Bar chart – but horizontal this time, which is how some computer packages produce them.

2.7 Frame 2.6 represents some results. Is there any way of knowing what they are about?

There is no way of knowing – the diagram needs to be properly labelled to tell you.

2.8 One principle in illustrating results is to give the diagram a ....

heading or title

2.9 The diagram in Frame 2.6 depicts the composition of cows' milk by weight.
88% is water
  3% is protein
  4% is fat
  5% is carbohydrate

Besides labelling the heading what else should be labelled?

The various sections

2.10 Pie chart or pie diagram

A *pie chart*, or *pie diagram*, provides a useful means of displaying data which are in the form of numbers falling within subgroups of an overall group or population. More than one such diagram can also be used to give a comparison between such groupings, at different times, say. When this is done, the *areas* of the pie charts can be made proportional to the numbers of individuals or items in the groups being compared. Note the distortion that results from making the linear measurements proportional to group size in this or any other two-dimensional representation of data. The example in the figure illustrates this type of diagram. The data (real) are for 569 mothers in one hospital, and give information on the normal practice for that hospital in terms of numbers of episiotomies performed. Further subgroups show the degree of perineal damage caused by the deliveries.

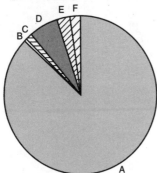

Key:
A – 495 (861) – Episiotomy without extension
B – 3 (1%) – Episiotomy + lacerations
C – 9 (2%) – Episiotomy + 3-degree tear
D – 35 (6%) – Intact perineum
E – 15 (3%) – Degree-1 tear
F – 12 (2%) – Degree-2 tear
569

Classification of 569 mothers under normal practice in one hospital by episiotomy or not and, further, by degree of perineal damage.

Results reported by R. F. Harrison, M. Brennan, P. M. North, J. V. Reed and E. A. Wickham 1984 British Medical Journal 288: 1971–1975.

This diagram has 2 further labels besides the heading and components. What are they?

The authors and the date

2.11 One of the principles of presenting data is to label fully. What should be labelled:
(1)   (2)   (3)   (4)

Heading, components author, date

2.12 To recap, what are the 4 main ways of presenting diagrammatically data which are qualitative?

Pie diagram, pictogram, bar chart and proportional bar chart

2.13 Besides being *fully labelled*, or self-explanatory, diagrams must be easy to understand. They should be as simple as possible, and not over-crowded with information. Look at the .... below. How would you improve it?

pie diagram
There is too much information in one diagram. A possible approach is to split it into two. This could be for males and females separately, or for practising and retired doctors separately.

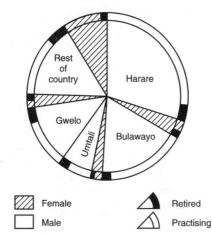

Areas in which doctors in Zimbabwe were practising (or are retired), showing sex. Data collected by Professor W. F. Ross, 1967 (but not presented like this!).

2.14 *Simplicity* is the second principle in presenting results. A good diagram will save a lot of words in the text. The diagram in Frame 2.10 is/is not a simple diagram because it would/would not save a lot of words in the text.

is
would

2.15 What may be described as the first 2 principles in depicting data?

Full labelling
Simplicity

2.16 There is a third – *honesty*. This does not mean just telling the truth but also the whole truth and nothing but the truth. There must be no attempt to mislead and justice must be seen to be done.
A manufacturer of a hair shampoo, 'Coo', gave free samples to 10 film stars. One lost the sample and the other 9 used theirs.
The manufacturer claims '*9 out of 10 film stars use Coo shampoo*'. Is he right?

If you *say yes*:
The slogan is dishonest and misleading although it does contain the truth in some sense.
If you *say no*:
You are not gullible. In reality the truth has been distorted by not providing the full information.

The inherent danger here has been set in the context of advertising, where there is clearly scope (hopefully usually avoided) for misrepresentation. But the dangers are also there in the medical context. Imagine, for example, the temptation for a clinician who fervently believes in some new treatment, in comparison with a standard one with which it is being compared.

2.17 How can you be dishonest with proportions and ratios, etc.?

By failing to record the total number considered

2.18 The same principles of presentation apply to quantitative data and moreover it is easier to be dishonest with that type of data. Apart from honesty, what other principles are involved in illustrating data?

Full labelling and simplicity

2.19 One of the reasons for diagrammatic presentation of data is to make the points clearer. What is the other?

To save words

2.20	What methods do you know for illustrating counts?	Pie diagram Bar chart Proportional bar chart Pictogram
2.21	Why would you use these methods?	To save words and make the points clear
2.22	To what principles would you adhere?	Full labelling, simplicity and honesty
2.23	**Practical example** Use a proportional bar chart to present the data in Frame 1.9.	See page 251.

SUMMARY

Hopefully, your example is fully labelled and is as simple as possible. Honesty is the other criterion, but this will be followed up further in the next chapter.

To present qualitative data diagrammatically, pie diagrams, pictograms, bar charts and proportional bar charts are used. They are intended to save words and make points clearer.

3. Illustrating measurements

INTRODUCTION

Quantitative results are generally more cumbersome than qualitative ones to represent diagrammatically. It is easier to represent sheep and goats than to distinguish diagrammatically between a 100 kg sheep and a 120 kg sheep.

3.1 *Birth-weights in kg of babies of mothers found to be suffering from diabetes mellitus* (fictitious data):

2.92	3.71	4.05
3.23	3.91	4.14
3.23	3.91	4.28
3.46	3.91	4.82

What kind of data are these?

Quantitative

3.2 The characteristic which is varying is called, not surprisingly, the *variable*. What is the variable in the last frame?

The birth-weight of babies of diabetic mothers

3.3 Such results as in Frame 3.1, but from large samples, are grouped before illustration. See below for a possible grouping of the data from the small sample in Frame 3.1. Is there more information in the data after grouping?

No. For example, no distinction is made now between the 3.23 kg and 3.46 kg birth weights.

Data from Frame 3.1 grouped:

Interval (kg)	Frequency
2.0–	0
2.5–	1
3.0–	3
3.5–	4
4.0–	3
4.5–	1
5.0–	0

The intervals have been set out in this way to emphasise that they represent '2.0 kg up to, but not including, 2.5 kg; from 2.5 kg up to, but not including, 3.0 kg', and so on (to avoid ambiguity at

3.3 *cont'd*
the boundaries). An alternative
representation for these data would
have been '2.00–2.49, 2.50–2.99' and so
on.

3.4 The price to pay for being able to
illustrate measurement is loss of some
information. The number in each group is
called the *frequency* of that group.
What is the frequency in the group   4
3.50–3.99 kg in the last frame?

3.5 All the frequencies considered together
form the *frequency distribution*. The
frequency distribution in Frame 3.3 is 0,
1, 3, 4, 3, 1, 0. What is the frequency
distribution below?

*Birth-weight in kg of 16 babies of normal
mothers* (fictitious data):

1.47	2.94	3.09	3.60
2.24	2.95	3.15	4.22
2.27	2.95	3.40	4.25
2.84	3.01	3.43	4.59

The above data can be grouped as
follows:

Interval (kg)	Frequency
0.5–	0
1.0–	1
1.5–	0
2.0–	2
2.5–	4
3.0–	5
3.5–	1
4.0–	2
4.5–	1
5.0–	0

According to this grouping the frequency   0, 1, 0, 2, 4, 5, 1, 2, 1, 0
distribution is what?

3.6 What is the variable in the last   The birth-weight of babies
frame?   of normal mothers

3.7 Why is haemoglobin level a variable?   Because it varies

3.8 Having grouped the data we can present them more easily in a diagram. Consider the diagram below depicting the results from Frame 3.3.

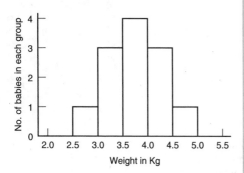

3.9 This method of illustration is called a *histogram*. Instead of 'No. of babies in each group' we could write

....

Frequency

In fact, we have to be rather careful about how we label the histogram. Since it is the *areas* of the rectangles in the histogram that correspond to the *frequencies* it is only valid to label the vertical axis as above when the class intervals are of equal width (for then, and only then, the *heights* of the rectangles are also proportional to the frequencies). In practice, it usually is the case that histograms are based on equal-width class intervals.

3.10 In your own words describe a histogram, and what it is used for.

A histogram is a method of presenting quantitative data diagrammatically. Along the horizontal axis is the variable under consideration. The histogram is a series of contiguous boxes standing side-by-side. The area of each box indicates the frequency in the group to which it corresponds. If the

3.10 *cont'd*

widths of the boxes are equal, then the heights of the boxes also indicate frequencies.

3.11 Draw a histogram to illustrate the data in Frame 3.5.

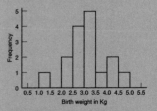

3.12 Another way of presenting data as in Frame 3.5 which is similar to a histogram, but which retains more of the detailed information, is as follows.

First, suppress the last decimal place in each case, yielding the following data:

1.4	2.9	3.0	3.6
2.2	2.9	3.1	4.2
2.2	2.9	3.4	4.2
2.8	3.0	3.4	4.5

They may then be listed as:

		Frequency	Cumulative frequency
O.B		0	0
1.A	4	1	1
1.B		0	1
2.A	2 2	2	3
2.B	8 9 9 9	4	7
3.A	0 0 1 4 4	5	[5]
3.B	6	1	4
4.A	2 2	2	3
4.B	5	1	1
5.A		0	0

This is called a stem-and-leaf diagram. The left-hand column is the stem. In this, A stands for 0, 1, 2, 3 or 4 and B stands for 5, 6, 7, 8 or 9. Hence 1.A means '1 point something (between 0 and 4)' and the 4 next to 1.A signifies 1.4. 2.A means '2 point something (between 0 and 4)' and the 2s next to 2.A signify 2.2 and 2.2, and so on. The numbers in the main body of the display, along the rows, are called the leaves. If these are properly

3.12   *cont'd*

lined up the shape of the display is like a
histogram on its side. Note that if we had
not had to suppress a decimal place, the
display would have retained the *full*
information in the data.

The frequency distribution is as we
saw it before (as we would expect).
The cumulative frequencies are
counted from each end, and
separated from the group containing
the middle observation, in size. (Note
that $7 + 5 + 4 = 16$, the total
frequency.) This is useful for finding
the median of the observed distribution.
We will discuss the median in
Chapter 6.

3.13   Another method of presenting measured
data is the *frequency polygon*. If the
midpoints of the tops of the boxes in the
histogram you drew earlier are joined by
a series of straight lines, you have the
equivalent frequency polygon. This type
of diagram can be useful when
comparing more than one distribution
(since histograms cannot easily be
superimposed), though it is not often
used.

Complete:

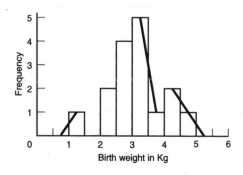

3.14   The boxes are not shown on a frequency
polygon, only the series of straight lines.
So what would the frequency polygon in
Frame 3.13 look like?

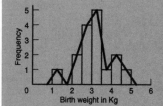

3.14 *cont'd*
If you wanted to show two frequency distributions such as Frames 3.3 and 3.5 on the same diagram, would you use 2 histograms or 2 frequency polygons?

2 frequency polygons, otherwise the boxes would overlap.

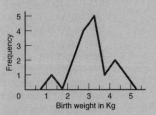

3.15 By convention, the frequency polygon is always continued until it meets the horizontal axis. Put another way, the frequency of the outside groups included in a frequency polygon is always

....

zero

3.16 30 Down's Syndrome children had the following distribution of I.Q.'s:

I.Q.	Frequency
60–69	3
70–79	5
80–89	11
90–99	7
100–109	4

Construct a frequency polygon to represent this frequency distribution.

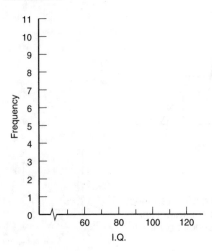

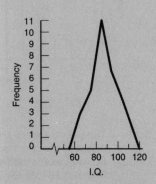

3.17 What are the 3 principles for good presentation of all results?

Full labelling; simplicity; honesty.

3.18 What is the commonest dishonest method used with qualitative data?

Not stating how many results were included in quoting percentages etc.

3.19 With quantitative data, cheating is very easy. We will warn you of 3 tricks to look out for. One such trick is to *suppress the zero*, e.g. *weight loss on 'Silfy' tablets*:

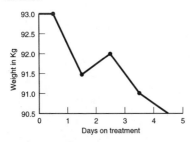

Re-sketch the diagram without suppressing the zero (i.e. mark 0 on both axes).

The weight loss does not look so impressive now, does it?

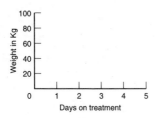

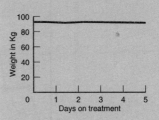

3.20 Although zero should often be shown on a diagram, sometimes the axis can be condensed as follows:

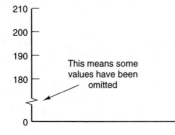

3.20   *cont'd*
Closely related to suppressing the zero
is the trick of *inflating or exaggerating
the scale*, e.g.

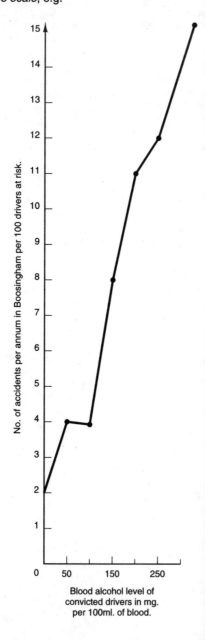

No. of accidents per annum in Boosingham per 100 drivers at risk.

Blood alcohol level of
convicted drivers in mg.
per 100ml. of blood.

3.20 *cont'd*
On a more reasonable scale this becomes:

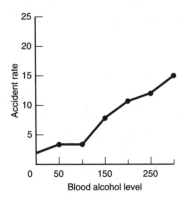

Blood alcohol level

What is a reasonable scale?

A reasonable scale is one which neither over-emphasises nor under-emphasises the evidence.

3.21 What is wrong with the diagram below? It shows the percentage of erythrocytes haemolysed in various concentrations of salt solution (Wintrobe's method).

It infers that more than 100% of the red cells survived at low concentrations. This is impossible.

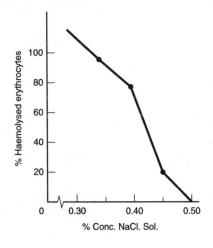

% Conc. NaCl. Sol.

3.22 The trick in Frame 3.21 is technically called *extrapolation* (extending the line beyond the actual results). In general, this is a dangerous thing to do, for we have no way of telling whether the results will follow the same pattern outside the range of values observed. In some cases, like the one here, they clearly cannot. What other 2 tricks do you know?

Suppressing the zero
Inflating the scale

3.23 What tricks have been employed in this diagram showing a patient's increase in haemoglobin level after therapy with the drug 'Ironical'?

All 3

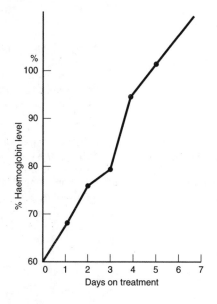

3.24 Which are the 3 commonest tricks used to illustrate quantitative data dishonestly?

Suppressing the zero
Inflating the scale
Extrapolation

3.25 What methods do you know for illustrating measurements?

Histograms, stem-and-leaf displays and frequency polygons

3.26 What methods do you know for illustrating counts?

Pie diagrams, bar charts, proportional bar charts and pictograms

3.27 The difference between a bar chart and a histogram is that the .... is used when data are measured and the .... is used for qualitative data. In the histogram the groups adjoin each other and the boxes abut each other, whereas with the bar chart the groups and the corresponding bars are usually ....

histogram
bar chart

separate

3.28 Ideally between 10 and 25 classes should be used in a histogram, depending on the number of observations.
How many are used here?

18

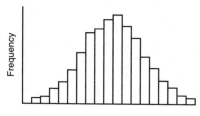

There is no hard and fast rule as to how many classes to use. If too many classes are used, most of the variability in the data is retained and the diagram is not helpful in summarising the pattern of the data. If too few classes are used, most of the variability is smoothed out altogether and the pattern in the data is simplified too much.

3.29 Sketch the frequency polygon that would be constructed from the histogram in the preceding frame – it would look like a curve.

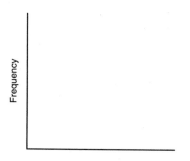

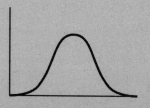

This diagram is the subject matter of the next chapter.

3.30　**Practical example**
Sketch the data from Frames 3.3 and
3.5 on the same diagram.

See page 251.

Comment.

Babies of diabetic mothers
seem to be bigger.

SUMMARY

Before presenting measurements the results are often grouped. The
number in each class is called the frequency. The collection of
frequencies in all the classes is called the frequency distribution. This
grouping makes illustration easier, but the price is some loss of detail.
Ideally, 10 to 25 different groups can be used, depending on the number
of observations, but no hard and fast rule can be given. The frequency
distribution is represented by a histogram or frequency polygon. When
2 or more frequency distributions are superimposed it is better to use the
corresponding number of frequency polygons.

Three dishonest tricks which may be used with quantitative data are
suppression of the zero, inflating the scale and extrapolation.

Honesty is a principle for presenting data. So is simplicity. Be on the
lookout for misleading or overly complicated presentations of data.

4. **The normal distribution**

INTRODUCTION

In the last chapter we imagined the approximation to the shape of a
curve constructed from a particular histogram. (Note that as the number
of classes gets larger (for large samples), and the class intervals smaller,
the frequency polygon corresponding to the histogram looks increasingly
like a curve.) Many biological and medical variables approximate to that
curve or can be transformed so that they do. Because it arises naturally
so often, and is used so commonly, it is important to understand it. (It is
not absolutely necessary to be able to remember its formula, however,
though even this is not too difficult to do.)

4.1	A factor which varies is called a	variable
4.2	In the pure sciences such as Physics and Chemistry there is not so much variability as in Biology and Medicine. One chemical carbon atom is much like another carbon atom – but when they are biologically arranged the effects can sometimes be very marked. How tall are you?	Your height is..........
4.3	We are 1.60 m and 1.80 m tall. Are you the same height as either of us?	Probably not, exactly
4.4	If your height is different from ours, which of us is abnormal?	Most likely none of us – at least as far as height is concerned!
4.5	Do you know more people over 1.85 m tall than under 1.85 m tall?	Probably not
4.6	Do you know more adults less than 1.50 m tall than over 1.50 m tall?	Probably not
4.7	The majority of adults are between 1.64 m and 1.74 m tall. Complete the schematic histogram below.	

4.7   *cont'd*

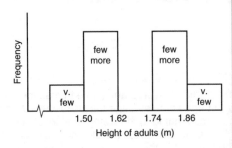

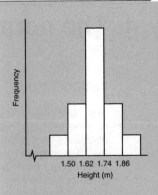

4.8   If we broke the results into many more
       small groups (e.g. 2 cm groups) and
       sketched the curve for adult males'
       heights, it could look like this:

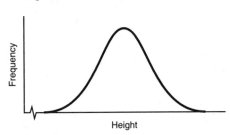

This is called the *normal distribution*.
It is shaped like a ....

It applies to qualitative or quantitative
data?

We describe the completed histogram
corresponding to Frame 4.8 and the
curve in Frame 4.9, as being *unimodal*,
as they have a single peak. It is quite
common with biological or medical data
to have a distribution which has two
peaks, and this is called *bimodal*.
Considering people's heights again, can
you think of a situation which might lead
to a bimodal distribution?

We shall need the idea of bimodality
again in Chapter 6.

4.9   A symmetrical curve is one with the two
       sides around the centre absolutely
       corresponding. The curve of the normal
       distribution is/is not symmetrical.

It is often described in
textbooks as being bell-
shaped.

Quantitative

If we have heights of both
adult males and adult
females in the distribution,
it is quite likely to be
bimodal. If we have
heights of adult males and
10-year-old boys in the
distribution it is very likely
to be bimodal.

It is.

4.9   *cont'd*

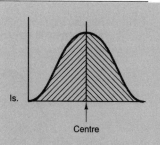

Is.

Centre

4.10   Which of the following are symmetrical?

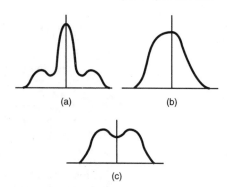

(a)   (b)

(c)   (a) and (c) are.

4.11   Describe the normal curve.   It is bell-shaped and
                                     symmetrical.

4.12   Relative to the base-line a convex
       surface is arched and a concave surface
       is hollow.

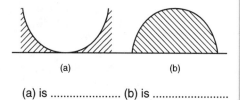

(a)   (b)

(a) is .... (b) is ....   concave, convex.

4.13   In this diagram indicate the part(s) which are convex and the part(s) which are concave.

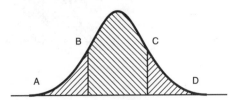

Between B and C it is arched or convex, otherwise it is hollow or concave.

4.14   The point where a convex section of a curve changes to a concave section is called a *point of inflection*.
How many points of inflection has a normal distribution curve?

2. They are B and C in the last frame.
You may wonder why we should be interested in such facts – surely they are of mathematical interest only. But it turns out (as we shall see later) that the position of the points of inflection on a normal curve have an interesting interpretation in terms of the amount of variability within the distribution.

4.15   In the diagram below, D is/is not a point of inflection?

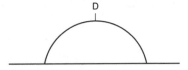

It is not.

4.16   Why?

The curve remains convex at point D.

4.17   We will meet the concept of point of inflection again later in the context of the normal distribution, and see what its particular interpretation is for that distribution.

4.18 For a variable to have a frequency distribution like the normal distribution the majority/minority have a measure near the middle and the majority/minority have measures near the extreme.

majority
minority

4.19 Is income distributed like the normal distribution?

No. The majority have a small wage and the minority a large wage.

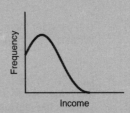

4.20 However, many variables based on living organisms can be described as being approximately normally distributed. Height is one example. Write down 3 others.
1. ....
2. ....
3. ....

I.Q., weight, bladder, capacity, haemoglobin level, body temperature, blood pressure, examination marks (usually), etc.

4.21 Describe the normal curve.

Symmetrical; bell-shaped; 2 points of inflection.

SUMMARY

Variation between individuals is a natural phenomenon, thank goodness. The fact that many variables either follow the normal distribution approximately or can easily be transformed to do so is very useful and enables variables to be used to answer questions, since the mathematics of the normal distribution is well known, and the features of it are extensively tabulated. The normal distribution is symmetrical and bell-shaped and has 2 points of inflection where the shape of the curve changes from being convex to concave.

What if variation between individuals does not approximate the normal distribution?

Statistical transformations are used to adjust the data so that the variable becomes more acceptable in terms of being normally, or nearly normally, distributed, for example. Square root, logarithmic (particularly), arcsin and probits are some commonly used statistical transformations.

An alternative approach to transforming the data to simulate normality, yet still providing a valid analysis of the data, is to use what are generally called nonparametric statistics, which we will meet in Chapter 21.

5. **Notation**

You are now to be introduced to symbols which will save a lot of words later. If your mathematics is such that you understand this chapter's summary you can skip the chapter.

5.1 n is used for the number of results.
What is n in Frame 3.1?

12

5.2   Usually x is used to represent an individual observation of a variable X.
What is the last x in Frame 3.1?

4.82 kg
Note the difference here between the variable X (weight) and a particular value x (in this case 4.82) of X.

5.3   If we have two results for each patient, e.g. a height and a weight, we usually call one x and one y (corresponding to the variables X and Y).
X and Y then represent two factors which vary or are ....

variables
Again, we distinguish between the variables, X and Y (height and weight), and observed values of those variables, x and y respectively.

5.4   How many values of X are there in any observed set of results, in general?

n

5.5 Σ is capital 'S' in Greek. It is pronounced 'sigma'. Σ means *add together* all the results. (So Σ is just shorthand for *add together*.)
What does Σ (1, 2, 2, 3) equal?

8

5.6 Σx means add together all the observed values x of X. It is pronounced
.... x.
What is Σx for the 5 following fictitious haemoglobin levels?

80, 90, 100, 110, 120

sigma

500

5.7 Below are corresponding values of X and Y for 5 students. X is haemoglobin level and Y is intelligence quotient, for example. n in each case equals ....

5

$\sum y$ equals ....

550

X: 80, 90, 100, 110, 120
Y: 80, 90, 100, 110, 170

5.8 What do $\frac{\sum x}{n}$ and $\frac{\sum y}{n}$ equal in the previous frame?

$\frac{\sum x}{n} = \frac{500}{5} = 100$

$\frac{\sum y}{n} = \frac{550}{5} = 110$

5.9 $\frac{\sum x}{n}$ is the average of the observed values x of the X variable, or the average of x, for short.

Its symbol is $\overline{x}$, called x bar.

What is the result $\frac{\sum y}{n}$ called?

The average of y, or $\overline{y}$, or y bar.

5.10 The average in statistical jargon is usually called the *mean*.
$\overline{y}$ is the .... of all the y.

mean

To be precise, this is the *arithmetic mean*. (There is another type of mean – the *geometric mean* – which is not used so much, but is appropriate in certain situations where a product of numbers is more meaningful than a sum of numbers. This is defined as the nth root of the product of n observations.)

5.11 $\overline{x}$ in Frame 5.6 = 100.

What does $\sqrt{\overline{x}}$ equal?

10

5.12 If 4 values of X are 2, 4, 6, 8, which symbol equals 4?

$n = 4$

Which symbol equals 5?

$\overline{x} = 5$

Which symbol equals 20?

$\sum x = 20$

5.13 When you see a capital sigma you do what?

Add the results together.

5.14 Sometimes we will want the results to be squared before adding.
We then write $\Sigma(x^2)$ or $\Sigma(y^2)$, or often just

Σx^2 or Σy^2 for short.

If Y is 1, 2, 2, 3, then
$\Sigma(y^2) = $ ....

$1 + 4 + 4 + 9 = 18$

You perform the task in brackets first; that is what the brackets mean. In fact this is often simply written as Σy^2. But note that this is *not* the same as $(\Sigma y)^2$.

5.15 $(x - \bar{x})$ means what?

An individual result minus the mean of the observed results.

5.16 $(x - \bar{x})$ is called *the deviation from the mean* (corresponding to the observation x). What is the last value of the deviation from the mean in Frame 5.6?

$120 - 100 = + 20$

5.17 It is a rule that you perform the task shown in brackets first.

What is $\Sigma(y - \bar{y})$ in Frame 5.6?

$(-20) + (-10) + (0) + (+10) + (+20) = 0$
Note that here the brackets are essential. $\Sigma y - \bar{y}$ would be quite different.

5.18 $\bar{y}$ in Frame 5.7 is 110.
What is $\Sigma(y - \bar{y})$ in that frame?

0

5.19 $\Sigma(x - \bar{x})$ and, of course, $\Sigma(y - \bar{y})$ always equal zero. In words, ...
........................equals zero.

the sum of the deviations from the mean
(If you are not convinced that it necessarily always equals zero, you may like to work through the algebra – if you are that way inclined – to assure yourself that this is so. For example,

5.19 *cont'd*	$\Sigma(x - \bar{x}) = \Sigma(x - \frac{\Sigma x}{n}) =$
	$\Sigma x - \Sigma(\frac{\Sigma x}{n}) = \Sigma x - \frac{n\Sigma x}{n}$
	$= 0.)$

5.20   In algebra xy equals a value x of X multiplied by its corresponding value y of Y. If X has the values 1, 2, 3 while the 3 corresponding values for Y are 1, 3, 4 the 3 values xy of XY are ...., ..., ..., and $\Sigma(xy) =$ ....

$1 \times 1 = 1$ $2 \times 3 = 6$
$3 \times 4 = 12$
$\Sigma(xy) = 1 + 6 + 12 = 19$

5.21   Remember, always perform the task in brackets first. If X has the values 1, 2, 2, 3, then $\bar{x}$ equals ...., and $\Sigma(x - \bar{x})^2$ equals ....

$2, (-1)^2 + (0)^2 + (0)^2 + (+1)^2 = 2$
Remember a negative number squared gives a positive answer.

5.22   If Y has the values 0, 2, 3, 3, then $\bar{y}$ equals ....
and $\Sigma(y - \bar{y})^2$ equals ....

2
6

5.23   Meanwhile $\Sigma(y - \bar{y}) =$ ....

0, as always

5.24   If Y has the values 0, 2, 3, 3,
$\Sigma y =$ ....
$\Sigma(y^2) =$ ....

8
22

5.25   Do you think $(\Sigma y)^2$ in the last frame equals
(A) 22
or (B) 64
or (C) any other answer?

If you say A – go to Frame 5.26.
If you say B – go to Frame 5.27.
If you say C – go to Frame 5.26.

5.26   You are incorrect.
$\Sigma(y^2)$ is not the same as $(\Sigma y)^2$.
In $\Sigma(y^2)$ you square and then add, while in $(\Sigma y)^2$ you add the results and then square your answer; (remember, perform the task inside the brackets first).

If y has the values 0, 1, 2,
$\Sigma(y^2)$ equals .... + ... + ...,
which equals 5,

$0 + 1 + 4$

$(\Sigma y)^2$ equals (........ + ... + ...)^2, which equals 9.

$(0 + 1 + 2)^2$

5.27   You know the difference between $\Sigma(y^2)$ and $(\Sigma y)^2$.

If X has the values 0, 1, 2 and Y has the values 1, 2, 3,
$(\Sigma x)(\Sigma y) = $ ...., and

$\Sigma(xy) = $ ....

$(\Sigma x)(\Sigma y) = 3 \times 6 = 18$

$\Sigma(xy) = 0 + 2 + 6 = 8$

5.28   That is all the notation you need to know throughout this book.

To revise it,

where X equals 1, 2, 4, 5 and Y equals 0, 0, 2, 2,

n in both cases equals	....	4
Σx	equals	12
Σy	equals	4
$\bar{x}$	equals	3
$\bar{y}$	equals	1
$\Sigma(x^2)$	equals	46
$(\Sigma x)^2$	equals	144
$\Sigma(xy)$	equals	18
$(\Sigma x)(\Sigma y)$	equals	48
$\Sigma(x - \bar{x})$	equals	0, of course
$\Sigma(y - \bar{y})^2$	equals	4

5.29   **Practical example**
Write down any 10 different values for X (i.e. $n = 10$) and substitute them in the table following. Using these numbers calculate in the spaces provided:

(a) $\dfrac{\Sigma(x - \bar{x})^2}{n - 1}$ =

(b) $\dfrac{\Sigma(x^2) - \dfrac{(\Sigma x)^2}{n}}{n - 1}$ =

The two answers should be equal.

5.29   *cont'd*

x	$(x - \bar{x})$	$(x - \bar{x})^2$	x	x^2
1				
2				
3				
4				
5				
6				
7				
8				
9				
10				

$\Sigma(x) =$ $\bar{x} =$	$\Sigma(x - \bar{x}) = 0$	$\Sigma(x - \bar{x})^2 =$	$\Sigma(x) =$ again	$\Sigma(x^2) =$

Therefore $\dfrac{\Sigma(x - \bar{x})^2}{n - 1}$ =

See page 252 for a worked example.

and $\dfrac{\Sigma(x^2) - \dfrac{(\Sigma x)^2}{n}}{n - 1}$ =

Are these two answers equal?

Yes, if the arithmetic is correct.

SUMMARY

n is the number of results recorded.

X and Y are variables and x and y, respectively, are the individual observations of those variables.

Σ (capital sigma) is the summation sign and means 'add together'.

$\bar{x} = \dfrac{\Sigma x}{n}$ is the mean (the arithmetic mean).

$(x - \bar{x})$ is a deviation from the mean.

$\Sigma(x - \bar{x})$ always equals 0.

Always work out the results in brackets first.

For example, $\Sigma(x^2)$ is the sum of the squares of the individual results. However, look out for when the brackets enclose the summation sign. For example, $(\Sigma x)^2$ is the sum of the individual results, all squared.
  Well done if you have got this far and understood it all. (If not, go back over the material again until you do.) These points will keep coming out throughout this book – rather like a rash. Honestly, this is all the mathematics and notation you need to understand.

6. **Measuring the middle**

INTRODUCTION

Rather than talk about a set of results in terms of all the individual values we can – and need to – summarise the information. We have already seen how to obtain diagrammatic summaries of data sets. We now begin to see how to obtain numerical summaries of them. To obtain helpful summaries of data sets we need to be able to describe 3 things, namely:

1. the *shape* of the distribution of the results (e.g. the normal distribution considered in Chapter 4) (note that diagrammatic summaries of data show us what the shape of their distribution is),

2. the *middle* of this distribution (considered in this chapter) and,

3. the *degree of variation*, or the *spread*, of the distribution (considered in the next chapter).

6.1   Describe the normal distribution.

It is symmetrical and bell-shaped with 2 points of inflection.

6.2   For the normal distribution the *mean* is in the middle.
What is the symbol for the mean of the variable X?

$\bar{X}$
(Note that $\bar{x}$ – which we have met already – is the mean of observed values x of the variable X.)

6.3   The mean is a measure of the middle of the distribution, as most of the results tend to lie about the mean. Is the 'range' of results a measure of the centre?

No. Note that it is possible to think of situations where most of the observations do not, in fact, lie about the mean (hence the choice of the word *usually* in this frame). For example, suppose we ask 50 third-year medical students how many issues of a particular monthly medical journal they read during the last calendar year. It is quite likely that there will be quite a large number who read 0, 1 or 2 issues, or 10, 11 or 12 issues, and relatively few or none who

| 6.3 | *cont'd* | read numbers of issues in the range 3 to 9. Yet the mean is most likely to fall in that mid-range. We will also see that the value of the mean can be pulled over (i.e. up or down) by a few extreme observations. |

| 6.4 | We are going to discuss 3 measures indicating the centre. One is the *mode*, another is the *median*, and the other is the .... | mean |

| 6.5 | If results are listed in order of size they are called an *array*. An examination list in alphabetical order is/is not an array. | It is not – unless the Aarons are at the top of the class and Zvakanakas at the bottom, etc.! |

| 6.6 | Are the results given in Frame 5.6 an array? | Yes |

| 6.7 | Do the results need to be arrayed before the mean is calculated? | No |

| 6.8 | The median is *the middle value in an array*. (If there are an even number of values in an array, the median is the mean of the two middle values.) What percentage of values (apart from the median itself) fall at or below the median in an array? | Half = 50% (The median is the value which cuts the distribution (array) into two equal parts.) |

| 6.9 | The results quoted in Frame 5.7 are repeated here: |

| X | 80, | 90, | 100, | 110, | 120 |
| Y | 80, | 90, | 100, | 110, | 170 |

What are the 2 values of the median?

100 – the same in each array

| 6.10 | The extreme value, 170, does not affect the median. Are the means in both distributions the same? | No $\bar{x}$ is 100 $\bar{y}$ is 110 |

6.11	Not only do the extreme values affect the mean but an extreme value has a greater/lesser effect than a value near to the middle.	greater
6.12	When we are interested in whether cases fall in the upper or lower half of the distribution, and are not particularly interested in how far they are from the central point, we use the median/the mean.	The median. In fact, as 50% lie below the median, the median can also be called 'the 50 percentile'.
6.13	The mean uses all the information available. Does the median?	No. In that sense, it is not such a reliable measure. The result 170 does not affect it. (So in cases where there are extreme values, we may feel that the median is, in fact, in some sense the more reliable measure, even though it does not use all the information.)
6.14	Which is easier to calculate, the median or the mean?	The median, especially if the results are already arrayed.
6.15	Choosing between the median and the mean, where applicable, we know: The .... is more reliable and is, in fact, usually used.	mean ('More reliable' is used here in the sense of using all the available information.)
	The .... is easier to calculate than the	median mean
	The .... is not affected by extreme values.	median
	To calculate the .... you need to array the results first.	median
6.16	Are these sedimentation rates an array? 7, 13, 11, 15, 10, 20.	No
6.17	What is the value of n in the previous frame?	6

6.18 So far, when we have calculated the median, *n* has been an odd number so that there has only been one middle value.
Is *n* odd or even in Frame 6.16?

Even

6.19 When *n* is even the median is the average, or mean, of the middle two values. What is the median in Frame 6.16?
(Hint: array the results first.)

12. The average of 11 and 13.

6.20 Consider the following representation (bar diagram) of a set of counts.

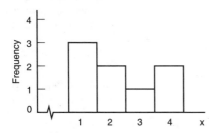

What is the distribution of the *x* values? *X* takes the values (1, 1, 1, 2, 2, 3, 4, 4) above.

The distribution is 1, 1, 1, 2, 2, 3, 4, 4.

What is the mean value?

Mean $= \dfrac{18}{8} = 2^{1}/_{4}$

What is the value of the median?

Median = 2

6.21 The mode is the value which occurs most frequently in a distribution. What is the mode in the last frame?

1
Note that the mean, median and mode are *not* the same (or even nearly the same) in this distribution. This should not surprise us, since the distribution is not symmetrical.

6.22 In the distribution represented by the diagram below, the mode, median and mean are/are not the same.

are
The distribution is 0, 1, 1, 1, 2, 2, 2, 2, 2, 3, 3, 3, 4.

6.22   *cont'd*

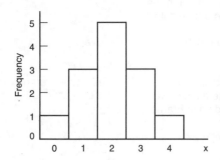

6.23   What are the values of the median, the mode and the mean in this normal distribution?

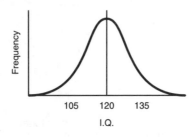

120
All the measures of the middle are always equal in the normal distribution.

6.24   The normal distribution is bell-shaped and symmetrical about the ...., ..., and ....

mean
median, mode

6.25   The .... and .... are easier to calculate than the .... if the results are arrayed.

mode, median
mean

6.26   What is the mode?

The value occurring most frequently

6.27   Some camels can be said to be bimodal!! Why?

Because they have 2 modes or humps.

6.28   The mode is the least valuable measure of the middle. When a variable approximates to the normal distribution the mean is the most useful measure of

Note that the modes in a bimodal distribution may not be of equal size, but because they are modes

6.28 *cont'd*

the middle. However, sometimes in research one comes upon a distribution with two modes. This is a helpful sign that two groups of dissimilar subjects are mixed together, i.e. that the group is probably heterogeneous. For example, the main groups of anaemias are macrocytic (with big cells) and microcytic (with small cells). Sketch the distribution of cell size in anaemias.

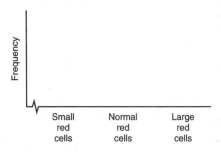

Distribution of cell size in all cases of anaemia.

locally (e.g. if the 'hump' for macrocytic anaemias had been slightly higher than that for microcytic anaemias) the distribution is still referred to as bimodal, and having 2 modes.

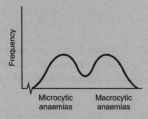

Note also that if in a bimodal distribution just the mean or the median is calculated, and no diagram of the data is inspected, you would miss the bimodal nature of the distribution.

6.29 The most reliable measure of the centre of a distribution which is at least approximately like a normal distribution is the .... It is/is not the only measure of the middle which uses all the information.

mean
Is (and it is in this sense that we mean 'reliable').

6.30 But if we wish to know the most typical value, then we would use the ....; or if we wish to know whether cases fall in the upper half or the lower half, then the .... is used; otherwise it is best to calculate the ....

But note that the mean can be badly affected by extreme observations. So if we are dealing with a highly skewed (asymmetrical) distribution it is better to use the ....

mode

median
mean

median

6.31 In this array:

1, 2, 3, 3, 4, 5, 10, 12

6.31	*cont'd*	
	3 is the value of the	mode
	5 is the value of the	mean
	and .... is the value of the	$3\frac{1}{2}$ median

6.32 We are now in a position to return to thinking about diagrammatic representations of data and to see how to produce 'box-and-whisker plots', or 'boxplots' for short. We will see that these are very attractive as simple diagrammatic summaries of observed data distributions.

6.33 Let us return to the data of Frame 3.5 (birth weights in kg of 16 babies of normal mothers).
What is the median of this data set?

The median is

$$\frac{3.01 + 3.09}{2} = 3.05$$

6.34 We now need to compute the *quartiles* of the distribution. The median splits the distribution into two equal parts. The quartiles split those two equal parts into two further equal parts.
How could you describe the median and the two quartiles in relation to an observed distribution?

They divide the set of values into four equal parts.

6.35 How would you compute the quartiles for the data in Frame 3.5?

Treat the values on either side of the median as two separate arrays. Then find the median of each of those arrays. These are then the quartiles.

6.36 What are the quartiles of the data in Frame 3.5?

Lower quartile =

$$\frac{2.84 + 2.94}{2} = 2.89$$

Upper quartile =

$$\frac{3.43 + 3.60}{2} = 3.515$$

6.37	What do you think the quartiles are, expressed as percentiles?	25 percentile and 75 percentile
6.38	What are the minimum and maximum values of the observed distribution?	1.47, 4.59

6.39   The box-and-whisker (boxplot) plot for the observed distribution is as follows:

0	1	2	3	4	5

Weight in Kg

The box provides a summary of the central part of the distribution. The lines emanating from the box are the 'whiskers'.

6.40	To what values in the distribution do the 3 vertical lines in the box correspond?	The lower quartile, the median and the upper quartile respectively, working from left to right
6.41	To what values in the distribution do the endpoints of the whiskers correspond?	The minimum and maximum values
6.42	What do you think the position of the middle vertical line in the box of the box-and-whisker plot (boxplot) might tell you about the shape of the distribution?	If the line is in the centre of the box it indicates that the central part of the distribution, at least, is symmetrical. If the line is off-centre it suggests that the central part of the distribution is asymmetrical, or skewed.
6.43	The boxplot is a very simple diagram conveying a lot of very useful information about the distribution of a set of observations. Try to suggest a way in which it might be especially useful, compared with a histogram.	It can be very useful to plot a number of boxplots together on the same page, and the same horizontal axis and scale, when comparing related

6.43   *cont'd*

distributions (e.g. patients' blood pressures in different treatment groups at a particular point in time in a clinical trial; patients' blood pressures at different time points within a single treatment group in a clinical trial). The boxplots would be drawn one above the other.

SUMMARY

The 3 most useful measures of the middle are the mean, the median and the mode.

The mean, or average, of the variable X has the symbol $\bar{X}$ and is the most useful measure. (The mean of the observed values x of a variable X is $\bar{x}$.) But it is markedly affected by extreme values.

The median and mode are calculated after the results are placed in order of size in an array.

The median is the middle value in an array (or the average of the middle two values if n is even). It is usually used if we are particularly interested in whether cases fall in the upper or the lower half of the distribution, or if the distribution is very skewed.

As 50% of cases (excluding the median itself) fall at or below the median in an array, it can also be called the 50 percentile.

The mode is easy to distinguish, being the value which occurs most frequently. If a frequency distribution is bimodal it usually means that the group is not homogeneous and two very different groups are mixed together. (Note that in principle it is possible to have a multimodal distribution, with more than two modes, even.) In the normal distribution the mean, the median and the mode fall in the same place.

The median of an observed distribution and, by extension, the quartiles, can be used, together with the extreme values, to construct a box-and-whisker plot, or boxplot, which provides a simple diagrammatic summary of the distribution. Particular advantage can be gained by plotting a number of boxplots on the same page when comparing related sets of observations.

7. Measuring the variation

INTRODUCTION

So far we have summarised a set of results by describing the shape and the centre. In this chapter we discuss how to measure variation, or spread.

7.1 Below we have two normal distributions, each with the same mean. One set of results varies more than the other – it has a bigger scatter. Is it distribution A or distribution B?

Distribution A. The results in distribution B cluster more closely about the mean. A has more variation between results.

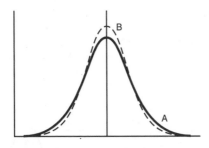

7.2 There were 3 measures of the centre discussed. What were they?

The mean, the mode and the median

7.3 Similarly there are 3 measures of variation. The first is the *range*. The range is the difference between the largest and smallest result. Does it use all the available information?

No

7.4 What is the range in Frame 5.6?

$120 - 80 = 40$

7.5 If 1, 2, 3, 3, 5, 9 is a distribution, 3 is the .... and the .... and 8 is the ....

median, mode
range

7.6 The mean is reliable because it uses all the information. Is the range a reliable measure of variation in the same sense?

No. It does not use all the information. (However, when we are dealing with a very small number of observations, it may be the most sensible measure to use.)

7.7

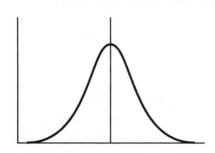

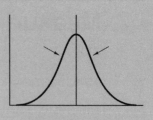

Mark the points of inflection above.

7.8 In the previous frame draw a horizontal line joining the points of inflection. This length can be used as a measure of variation. If the results are very scattered the line is longer/shorter than if they cluster around the mean.

longer

7.9 In fact the length of this horizontal line from a point of inflection to the *mean* in a normal distribution is called the *standard deviation*. It is a very useful measure of variation. Draw in the standard deviation below.

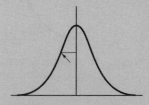

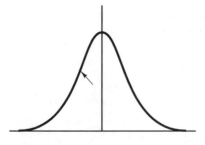

Note, then, that this is the practical interpretation of the points of inflection in a normal distribution, in terms of a measure of variation, that we had been anticipating from Chapter 4.

7.10 The standard deviation is often given the symbol *s*. We need to calculate this value. We know it does not equal $\sum(x - \bar{x})$.
Why?

This value always equals 0.

7.11 Therefore, $\dfrac{\sum(x - \bar{x})}{n}$ is also equal to

What we have done here is to ensure, by squaring,

7.11 *cont'd*
0, so cannot be used as a measure of variation either. In fact, *s* has a slightly more complicated formula than this. It is:

$$s = \sqrt{\frac{\Sigma(x - \bar{x})^2}{n - 1}}$$

s^2 is the other measure of variation and is called the sample *variance*.

Give the formula for the variance:

$$s^2 =$$

that each deviation, $(x - \bar{x})$ (squared to give $(x - \bar{x})^2$), contributes a positive term to the formula, whether $(x - \bar{x})$ itself is positive or negative.

$$\frac{\Sigma(x - \bar{x})^2}{n - 1}$$

7.12 You have met the $\Sigma(x - \bar{x})^2$ part before at the end of Chapter 5 and you know that *n* is what?

The number of results
In this formula we have $n - 1$, rather than n, and $n - 1$ is called the number of *degrees of freedom*.

7.13 If observed values *x* of *X* are 0, 1, 2, 2, 5, then $\bar{x} =$ .... and

$$\Sigma(x - \bar{x})^2 = \text{.....................}$$

$$\bar{x} = \frac{10}{5} = 2$$

$$\Sigma(x - \bar{x})^2 = 4 + 1 + 0 + 0 + 9 = 14$$

7.14 Hence, if values of *X* are 0, 1, 2, 2, 5, then $\Sigma(x - \bar{x})^2 = 14$ and $s^2 =$

$$s^2 = \frac{14}{4} = 3^1/_2$$

7.15 $(x - \bar{x})$ is called ....
(words)

the deviation from the mean

7.16 State the formula, $s^2 = \dfrac{\Sigma(x - \bar{x})^2}{n - 1}$, in words.

The variance is the sum of the squares of the deviations from the mean divided by one less than the number of results.

7.17 $\sqrt{\dfrac{\Sigma(x - \bar{x})^2}{n - 1}}$ is the formula for *s*,

which is called what?

The standard deviation

7.18 Complete this calculation of the standard deviation from Frame 5.6 by deciding the values of a, b, c, d, s^2 and s. ($x = 100$.)

x	$(x - \bar{x})$	$(x - \bar{x})^2$
80	-20	400
90	(a)	(b)
100	0	0
110	$+10$	100
120	$+20$	400

$a = -10$
$b = 100$
$c = 1000$
$d = n - 1 = 4$

$$\sum(x - \bar{x})^2 = (c)$$

$$\frac{\sum(x - \bar{x})^2}{n - 1} = \frac{(c)}{(d)} = s^2 =$$

$s^2 = 250$

$$s =$$

$s = \sqrt{250}$

7.19 It is easier to calculate the range than the standard deviation. Why is the standard deviation a better measure?

It uses all the information.

7.20 What is the symbol for the standard deviation and what is its formula?

$$s = \sqrt{\frac{\sum(x - \bar{x})^2}{n - 1}}$$

7.21 s^2 is the ....

What is its formula?

variance

$$s^2 = \frac{\sum(x - \bar{x})^2}{n - 1}$$

Note that the units in which variance is measured are the square of the units of the original observations. The units of standard deviation are the same as the original units.

7.22 If X takes the values 1, 1, 2, 3, 3:

What is the range?
What is $\bar{x}$?
What is the value of the variance?
What is the value of the standard deviation?

range = 2
$\bar{x} = 2$

$$s^2 = \frac{[(1 - 2)^2 + (1 - 2)^2 + (2 - 2)^2 + (3 - 2)^2 + (3 - 2)^2]}{4}$$

7.22 *cont'd*

$$= \frac{(1^2 + 1^2 + 0 + 1^2 + 1^2)}{4} = 1$$

$$s = \sqrt{1} = 1$$

7.23 If X still takes the values 1, 1, 2, 3, 3:
What is $\Sigma(x^2)$?
What is $(\Sigma x)^2$?

$\Sigma(x^2) = 24$
$(\Sigma x)^2 = 10^2 = 100$

7.24 Then, what does $\dfrac{\Sigma(x^2) - \dfrac{(\Sigma x)^2}{n}}{n - 1}$ equal?

$\dfrac{24 - \dfrac{100}{5}}{4} = 1$

7.25 Hence, when X takes the values 1, 1, 2, 3, 3,

$$\frac{\Sigma(x - \bar{x})^2}{n - 1} = 1 \text{ (from Frame 7.22)}$$

and $\dfrac{\Sigma(x^2) - \dfrac{(\Sigma x)^2}{n}}{n - 1} = 1$ (from Frame 7.24).

In fact, whatever the distribution *it is always arithmetically true* that

$$\frac{\Sigma(x - \bar{x})^2}{n - 1} = \frac{\Sigma(x^2) - \dfrac{(\Sigma x)^2}{n}}{n - 1}$$

Therefore $\sqrt{\dfrac{\Sigma(x^2) - \dfrac{(\Sigma x)^2}{n}}{n - 1}}$ is another

formula for calculating .... Indeed, this is in general the most convenient formula for calculating s.

s, the standard deviation. In fact, you saw this to be so in the practical example in Frame 5.29.

7.26 Which of these, if any, is a correct formula for the standard deviation?

(d) and (g)

(a) $\sqrt{\dfrac{(\Sigma x - \bar{x})^2}{n - 1}}$

(a) has the summation sign inside the bracket.

7.26 *cont'd*

(b) $\sqrt{\dfrac{\Sigma(x - \bar{x})^2}{n}}$

(b) has not got the usual denominator.

(c) $\sqrt{\dfrac{(\Sigma x)^2 - \dfrac{\Sigma(x^2)}{n}}{n - 1}}$

(c) has both brackets in the wrong place.

(d) $\sqrt{\dfrac{(\Sigma x^2) - \dfrac{(\Sigma x)^2}{n}}{n - 1}}$

(e) $\sqrt{\dfrac{\Sigma(x - \bar{x})}{n - 1}}$

(e) omits the square.

(f) $\dfrac{\Sigma(x - \bar{x})^2}{n - 1}$

(f) omits the square root sign.

(g) $\sqrt{\dfrac{\Sigma(x - \bar{x})^2}{n - 1}}$

7.27 One formula for the standard deviation does not need to have the mean calculated first. What is it?

$\sqrt{\dfrac{\Sigma(x^2) - \dfrac{(\Sigma x)^2}{n}}{n - 1}}$

7.28 If the mean is a whole number, it is easier to use the formula

$\sqrt{\dfrac{\Sigma(x - \bar{x})^2}{n - 1}}$ for s.

If $\bar{x}$ was calculated to be 2.3816 it would be easier to use which formula?

The one not requiring the calculation of deviations from the mean,

i.e. $s = \sqrt{\dfrac{\Sigma(x^2) - \dfrac{(\Sigma x)^2}{n}}{n - 1}}$

Indeed, if in doubt, use this one anyway. You never lose much, in terms of effort, calculating the standard deviation in this way, and you often (in fact, usually) gain a lot. In any case, discussion of which formula to use is often redundant nowadays, since you will be carrying out your calculations on a computer, or a calculator with statistical facilities.

7.29 If X takes the values 2, 3, 3, 4, 5,

$\bar{x} = 3.4$

Complete the following table:

x	$x - \bar{x}$	$(x - \bar{x})^2$	x^2
2	-1.4		4
3	-0.4	0.16	9
3	-0.4	0.16	
4			16
5	$+1.6$	2.56	
$\Sigma x =$	$\Sigma(x - \bar{x}) = 0$	$\Sigma(x - \bar{x})^2 =$	$\Sigma x^2 =$

x	$x - \bar{x}$	$(x - \bar{x})^2$	x^2
2	-1.4	1.96	4
3	-0.4	0.16	9
3	-0.4	0.16	9
4	$+0.6$	0.36	16
5	$+1.6$	2.56	25
17	0	5.20	63

7.30 Hence the variance $= \dfrac{\Sigma(x - \bar{x})^2}{n - 1} =$

$\dfrac{5.20}{4} = 1.30$

and also the variance $= \dfrac{\Sigma(x^2) - \dfrac{(\Sigma x)^2}{n}}{n - 1} =$

The same,

$\dfrac{63 - \dfrac{17^2}{5}}{4} = 1.30$

7.31 Give the formula for the standard deviation without using the mean.

$s = \sqrt{\dfrac{\Sigma(x^2) - \dfrac{(\Sigma x)^2}{n}}{n - 1}}$

7.32 The standard deviation for I.Q. in a group of people is about 15. What is the variance for I.Q.?

About 225

7.33 A frequency distribution in a journal looks like this. Describe it as fully as possible.

Shape – normal.
Mean/median/mode = 100
Standard deviation = 10
Variance = 100
Range = 60
(But note that the theoretical normal distribution goes off to infinity in both directions but with very low tails in the frequency distribution curve.)

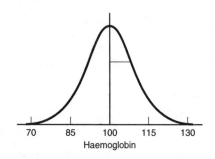

70	85	100	115	130

Haemoglobin

7.34 Like the ...., which measures the middle of a distribution, the standard deviation and variance use all the data. They are more reliable measures in that sense than the .... and .... which measure the middle, and the .... which measures variation.

mean

median, mode
range

7.35 State two formulae for the variance.

$$s^2 = \frac{\Sigma(x - \bar{x})^2}{n - 1}$$

$$= \frac{\Sigma(x^2) - \frac{(\Sigma x)^2}{n}}{n - 1}$$

7.36 In an examination you would probably be given any formulae which are harder' than these. However, the standard deviation and variance are so important that you could be expected to remember them. Can you?

Yes, we hope so. If not, it is worth going back through this chapter and making sure that you know them. Also, of course, the second formula is valid even when the mean *is* a whole number. So if you are in any doubt, use this formula all the time.

7.37 If the value of $\bar{x}$ is not a whole number, which formula would you use for the variance?

$$\frac{\Sigma(x^2) - \frac{(\Sigma x)^2}{n}}{n - 1}$$

7.38 If Y is the variable rather than X, what would be the formula for the standard deviation without using $\bar{y}$?

$$\frac{\Sigma(y^2) - \frac{(\Sigma y)^2}{n}}{n - 1}$$

7.39 One measure of variation does not use all the information. It is the ...., which is often used when the .... is used as the measure for the centre.

range
median

7.40 Sketch a normal distribution with mean 60, standard deviation 4 and range 24.

7.40   *cont'd*

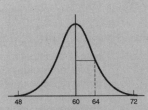

Note that the true range of a theoretical normal distribution is infinite.

7.41   In journals you often see written: 'the mean ± the standard deviation'. For example, 100 ± 15 for I.Q., seen in an article, indicates what?

That the mean I.Q. is 100 and the standard deviation is 15.
It is not necessarily good practice to do this without explicitly stating what the ± part is (i.e. the standard deviation). But the convention is now well established and recognised.

7.42   Another name for the 50 percentile is the
....

median

7.43   50% of results fall below the 50 percentile. 10% of results fall below the .... percentile and 95% below the .... percentile.

10
95

7.44   A child weighs less than the 3 percentile for his age group.
Comment.

The child is extremely light. 97% of the children are heavier. Percentiles are often used to measure how extreme a result is, particularly for heights and weights of children. *Q*% lie below the *Q* percentile.

7.45   **Practical example**
Results in reality are not so arithmetically convenient as in this programme. They are usually more like those in Frames 3.1 and 3.5. Calculate the mean and

See page 252.

7.45   *cont'd*
standard deviation in Frame 3.1 and
Frame 3.5. We will use the answers in
Chapter 17 when we test to see whether
babies of diabetic mothers are
significantly bigger than those of normal
mothers, so your efforts now will be put
to practical use later. In fact,
arithmetically you could perform
significance tests based on means
already, but we want you to *understand*
what you are doing first of all, because
the tests are then much more
interesting.

SUMMARY

Measures of variation are used to indicate the spread of a distribution.
The variance, s^2, and its square root, the standard deviation, s, are the
measures of choice; the range is occasionally used.

The range of the results is easy to calculate but has the same
disadvantage as the median and mode – that it is not a reliable
measurement in the sense that it does not use all the available
information. It is used as a measure of variation when the median is used
as a measure of the centre. The range is the difference between the
highest and lowest values. Q percentiles are values below which $Q\%$ of
the results fall. The formulae to calculate the variance are

$$\frac{\Sigma(x^2) - \dfrac{(\Sigma x)^2}{n}}{n - 1} \quad \text{and} \quad \frac{\Sigma(x - \bar{x})^2}{n - 1}$$

which are numerically identical.

The standard deviation in the normal distribution is the horizontal
measurement from the mean to a point of inflection and is the square
root of the variance.

8. What correlation means

INTRODUCTION

So far we have learned to describe qualitative data in terms of ratios and rates etc. and quantitative data in terms of the shape, middle and variation (spread) of the frequency distributions. When two or more different variables are measured on the same people (or animals, or other subjects) to see whether one is associated with the other (a common practice in medical research) we describe the results in terms of correlation.

8.1   Correlation does not mean causation. The probability of getting lung cancer and the number of cigarettes smoked have been shown to be correlated. Does this necessarily mean smoking causes lung cancer?

> No, not by itself. No more than lung cancer causes smoking. It does show, though, that there is an association between smoking and lung cancer.

8.2   Correlation means which of the following?
(a) association
(b) causation
(c) living with relatives!
(d) tied together
(e) acting in the same way

> (a)

8.3   Height and weight are correlated. Increase in weight is associated with increase/decrease in height.

> increase

8.4   When an increase in one variable is associated with an increase in another, correlation is said to be *positive*. A decrease in one variable associated with an increase in another is *negative* correlation. Size of shoe and size of hat are correlated how?

> Positively

8.5   Time spent in bed and time spent on studying are .... correlated.

> Negatively – unless you study in bed!

8.6   How are I.Q. of parent and I.Q. of child correlated?

> Positively

8.7	When two variables are considered simultaneously in terms of correlation, the information may be represented on a scatter diagram. What are the two variables in this scatter diagram?	*X* and *Y*

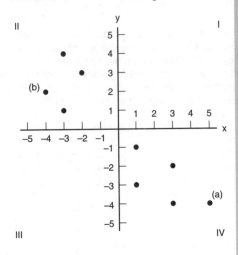

8.8	Each dot in the last frame is where a value of *X* corresponds to a value of *Y*. At point (a) *X* is +5 while *Y* is ....?	−4
8.9	At point (b) .... is positive and .... is negative.	*Y, X*
8.10	In the quadrant marked II, *X* is .... and *Y* is	negative positive
8.11	In quadrant I, *X* and *Y* are both positive; in quadrant III, *X* and *Y* are both negative. When most points lie in quadrants I and III the correlation is positive/negative.	positive
8.12	Which quadrants would contain most dots if correlation were negative?	II and IV
8.13	In Frame 8.7 correlation is	negative

8.14 When no correlation exists the dots in the .... occur roughly the same amount in all quadrants (like a non-specific rash).

scatter diagram

8.15 Draw quadrants in this scatter diagram.

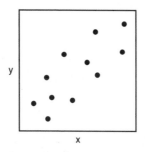

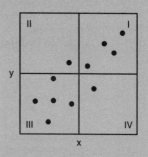

Is correlation positive or negative?

Positive

8.16 The quadrants are only aids and need not be shown. Manage without them and complete the following:

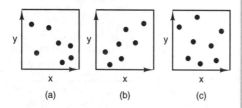

In (a) there is .... correlation
In (b) there is .... correlation
In (c) there is .... correlation

negative
positive
no

8.17 So far we have learned to describe the direction or the sign of the correlation. The magnitude of the correlation also has descriptive value. It is at its *maximum* when the points fall exactly on a slope so that they lie on a straight line. The more the points are scattered about the sloped line the less the correlation becomes, until when the points are scattered all over the place there is no correlation at all. It is not the steepness of the slope that determines

It is worth repeating the point about linearity here for emphasis. Correlation gives a measure of the amount of *linear* association between a pair of variables. This is often not appreciated.

8.17 *cont'd*
the degree of correlation but how close
the points are to a straight line. In fact
the steepness of the slope – its gradient
– is what regression is all about. Note
that correlation measures the degree of
linear association between a pair of
variables. It is possible for a pair of
variables to be strongly associated, but
not linearly, in which case there might be
no correlation.
Correlation is/is not greater in (a) than
(b).

is

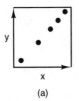
(a)

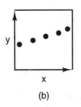
(b)

8.18 Correlation is at its maximum in which of
the following:
  (i) (a) only?
 (ii) (b) only?
(iii) both (a) and (b)?

Both (a) and (b), as in
both scatter diagrams
the points lie exactly on
a straight line. This is a
state of affairs which is
rarely met in reality.
In fact the regression is
greater in (a) because
the slope is steeper.
Remember, the
correlation coefficient
tells us nothing about
the gradient of the
slope.

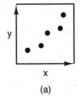
(a)

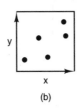
(b)

8.19 Put this information into a scatter
diagram and answer the questions.

X, Height of father (cm)	Y, Height of eldest adult son (cm)
168	173
173	175
175	178
180	178
185	180

8.19   *cont'd*

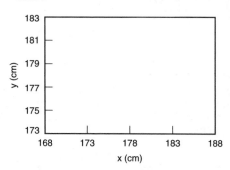

Is correlation present? If so, is it positive or negative?

Yes. Positive

Is it probably greater than in the diagram below?

Yes

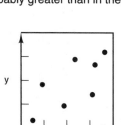

8.20   Correlation means ....

association (linear)

SUMMARY

Correlation means linear association. It can be positive, negative or non-existent. Positive correlation is where the variables tend to increase in size together. When two variables are involved a scatter diagram may be used to represent the data. With positive correlation the dots tend to lie in the upper right-hand and lower left-hand quadrants, while with negative correlation the dots tend to lie in the other two quadrants. There is no preponderance of dots in any quadrant where correlation does not exist. The magnitude of correlation is indicated by how closely the dots approximate to a straight line (i.e., how narrow the scatter is about an imaginary line), and not by their slope. If in fact the dots do approximate to a straight line which is sloped, it is then meaningful to talk about the gradient of the slope. This is one of the basic concepts of regression by which, for example, we can predict the value of one variable for a given value of the other. We will explore these ideas further in Chapter 19.

9. Measuring correlation

INTRODUCTION

You will learn here about two ways of measuring correlation. You would usually not be expected to remember these formulae (though you should understand the *form* of them), but having been given them you would be expected to be able to use them.

9.1   One measure of correlation is called the *Pearson correlation coefficient* and its symbol is '*r*'. (The full name is 'Pearson's product-moment correlation coefficient' – we will see why later.)

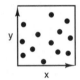

You would expect '*r*' to equal .... approximately here.

0

9.2   How are many variables approximately distributed?

Normally

9.3   In order to calculate '*r*' *and for the value to be meaningful* both variables involved, in theory, must be distributed normally. May '*r*' be calculated between height and weight?

Yes, if both are regarded as being approximately normally distributed (which is quite likely to be true).

9.4   Should '*r*' between I.Q. and income be calculated?
Their frequency distributions are given below.

No

Income does not follow the normal distribution shape.

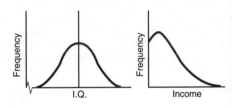

9.5 Complete this diagram with *r* taking its maximum absolute value, but negative, by adding two dots.

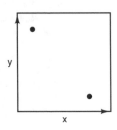

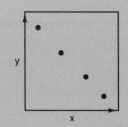

The dots lie in a straight line.

9.6 *r* is .... than its maximum value here and its sign is ....

less
positive

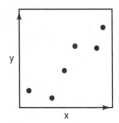

9.7 Give a formula for the standard deviation, *s*, of a set of observed values *x* of the variable *X* – without looking back to Chapter 7 if possible.

$$s = \sqrt{\frac{\sum(x - \bar{x})^2}{n - 1}}$$

or $\sqrt{\dfrac{\sum(x^2) - \dfrac{(\sum x)^2}{n}}{n - 1}}$

9.8 The denominator for *r* is

$$\sqrt{\frac{\sum(x - \bar{x})^2}{n - 1}} \times \sqrt{\frac{\sum(y - \bar{y})^2}{n - 1}},$$

which is what?

The form of this is the standard deviation of *x* multiplied by the standard deviation of *y*. Symbolically it is represented by $s_x s_y$.

9.9 Write $s_x s_y$ without using the means.

$$\sqrt{\frac{\sum(x^2) - \frac{(\sum x)^2}{n}}{n - 1}} \times \sqrt{\frac{\sum(y^2) - \frac{(\sum y)^2}{n}}{n - 1}}$$

9.10 Is $\sum(x - \bar{x})^2$ the same as $\sum(x - \bar{x})(x - \bar{x})$?

Yes

9.11 The numerator for r is $\dfrac{\Sigma(x - \bar{x})(y - \bar{y})}{n - 1}$

Comment.

It is very similar to the formula for the variance, only now with x and y involved, rather than just x or y. It is, incidentally, called the *covariance* for X and Y, denoted by s_{xy}. It is this that leads to the name of *product-moment correlation coefficient*, which we met at the beginning of this chapter.

9.12 As $\dfrac{\Sigma(x - \bar{x})^2}{n - 1} = \dfrac{\Sigma(x^2) - \dfrac{(\Sigma x)^2}{n}}{n - 1}$,

do you think

$$\frac{\Sigma(x - \bar{x})(y - \bar{y})}{n - 1} = \frac{\Sigma(xy) - \dfrac{(\Sigma x)(\Sigma y)}{n}}{n - 1} \,?$$

Yes, it does. (This can be easily confirmed by working through the algebra and summations.) Again, this leads to a simpler form for computations.

9.13 $r = \dfrac{\text{covariance of } X \text{ and } Y}{s_x s_y} = \dfrac{s_{xy}}{s_x s_y}$

So, without using means (as very rarely are both $\bar{x}$ and $\bar{y}$ whole numbers),

$r = ?$

$$r = \frac{\dfrac{\Sigma(xy) - \dfrac{(\Sigma x)(\Sigma y)}{n}}{n - 1}}{\sqrt{\dfrac{\Sigma(x^2) - \dfrac{(\Sigma x)^2}{n}}{n - 1}} \times \sqrt{\dfrac{\Sigma(y^2) - \dfrac{(\Sigma y)^2}{n}}{n - 1}}}$$

9.14 In fact the $n - 1$ term in the numerator can be cancelled with the

$\sqrt{n - 1} \times \sqrt{n - 1}$ in the denominator,

so that

$$r = \frac{\Sigma(xy) - \dfrac{(\Sigma x)(\Sigma y)}{n}}{\sqrt{\Sigma(x^2) - \dfrac{(\Sigma x)^2}{n}} \; \sqrt{\Sigma(y^2) - \dfrac{(\Sigma y)^2}{n}}}.$$

To what does n refer?

The number of X results or the number of Y results, i.e. the number of pairs of results (points on the scatter diagram).

9.15 This formula looks daunting but we will use it now to show that it is not too hard to implement. (For your convenience in the future it has been reproduced at the back of the book.) To use this formula you need/need not know the means of *x* and *y*.

need not
In fact, the formula is not all that daunting anyway, since each of the three parts of it has the same format, so once you have remembered one part of it you should be able to remember the whole thing.

9.16 We will use the formula to calculate the value for *r* in this scatter diagram.

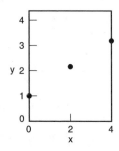

We expect here the sign of *r* to be .... and *r* to equal its maximum value.

positive

9.17 Transfer these three results to complete the table below.

x	y
0	(b)
(a)	2
4	3

$n = $ (c)

(a) = 2
(b) = 1
(c) = 3, the number of pairs of results

9.18 To use the formula for *r* we need to know

$\Sigma(xy)$, $\Sigma(x)$, $\Sigma(y)$, $\Sigma(x^2)$ and $\Sigma(y^2)$

(often written Σxy, Σx, Σy, Σx^2, Σy^2 for short, since there should be no possibility of ambiguity).

9.18 *cont'd*
Complete the following table:

(x)	(x²)	(y)	(y²)	(xy)
0	0	1	(b)	0
2	(a)	2	4	4
4	16	3	9	(c)
$\Sigma(x) = 6$	$\Sigma(x^2) = 20$	$\Sigma(y) = $ (d)	$\Sigma(y^2) = $ (e)	$\Sigma(xy) = $ (f)

(a) = 4
(b) = 1
(c) = 12
(d) = 6
(e) = 14
(f) = 16

9.19 Using the totals you have already calculated, i.e.

$n = 3$ $\qquad \Sigma(xy) = 16$

$\Sigma(x) = 6$ $\qquad \Sigma(x^2) = 20$

$\Sigma(y) = 6$ $\qquad \Sigma(y^2) = 14,$

what is the value of the numerator in calculating r?

$$\left[\text{Remember, it is given by:} \atop \Sigma(xy) - \frac{(\Sigma x)(\Sigma y)}{n}. \right]$$

$16 - \dfrac{6 \times 6}{3}$

$= 16 - 12 = 4$

9.20 What is the value of the denominator in calculating r?

$$\left[\text{Remember, this is given by:} \atop \sqrt{\Sigma(x^2) - \frac{(\Sigma x)^2}{n}} \ \sqrt{\Sigma(y^2) - \frac{(\Sigma y)^2}{n}}. \right]$$

$\sqrt{20 - \dfrac{6 \times 6}{3}} \times \sqrt{14 - \dfrac{6 \times 6}{3}}$

$= \sqrt{(20 - 12)} \times \sqrt{(14 - 12)}$

$= \sqrt{8} \times \sqrt{2} = \sqrt{16} = 4$

9.21 $\therefore$ r takes its maximum value, given by
....

$\dfrac{4}{4} = +1$ (from Frames

19.19 and 19.20)

9.22 If you ever calculated r to be 5, what would be your conclusion?

You have made an arithmetical error, because 1 is its maximum possible value.

9.23 What is the value of r here?

-1
This is the lowest possible value (or the maximum value of r in magnitude, but negative).

9.23 *cont'd*

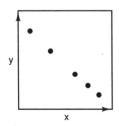

9.24 The Pearson correlation coefficient has a *sign* and a *numerical value*.

What do these signify?

The sign signifies the direction of the slope of the points and the numerical value signifies how closely the points lie to a straight line. Remember that the numerical value of the correlation coefficient tells us nothing about the slope of the line.

9.25 Guess which of the following 6 values for r is correct here.

$-0.1, \quad -0.5, \quad -1.0,$

$-0.9, \quad 0, \quad +0.9$

-0.9

9.26 You can use the formula to calculate r in the last frame by completing this table.

$\sum(x) = 11 \qquad \sum(y) = 13$

$\sum(x^2) = 31 \qquad \sum(y^2) = 41$

$\sum(xy) = 13 \qquad n = 6$

$$r = \frac{13 - \dfrac{11 \times 13}{6}}{\sqrt{\left[31 - \dfrac{11^2}{6}\right]} \ \sqrt{\left[41 - \dfrac{13^2}{6}\right]}}$$

9.26   *cont'd*

(x)	(x²)	(y)	(y²)	(xy)
0		4		
1		4		
1		2		
2		2		
3		1		
4		0		
Σ(x) =	Σ(x²) =	Σ(y) =	Σ(y²) =	Σ(xy) =

$n =$

∴ *r* approximately =

$$= \frac{13 - \frac{143}{6}}{\sqrt{(31 - 20.2)} \ \sqrt{(41 - 28.2)}}$$

$$\approx \frac{-11}{\sqrt{11} \times \sqrt{13}}$$

(≈ means approximately

equals) $\approx \dfrac{\sqrt{11}}{\sqrt{13}} \approx \dfrac{-3.3}{3.6} \approx -0.9$

9.27   *r* is the .... It is used for .... data for which it is reasonable to suppose that they are distributed..........

Pearson (product-moment) correlation coefficient, quantitative, normally

The other coefficient of correlation we are going to discuss in this book is *Spearman's rank order correlation coefficient*. Its symbol is ρ (rho). The formula, which you need not remember (though you may not find it especially difficult to do so), is

$$1 - \frac{6\Sigma(d^2)}{n(n^2 - 1)}$$

n is the same in both correlation coefficient formulae. What does it represent?

The number of pairs of results.

9.28   As the name 'rank order correlation coefficient' implies, ρ deals not with the actual results but with their rank order; if *n* is 6, and the best is ranked 1 or 1st, the worst would be ranked ....?

6 or 6th

9.29   Here are the fictitious 2nd M.B. marks for 5 candidates.
B was bottom in Anatomy and was ranked 5th or 5.

C is ranked .... in Anatomy.

3rd or 3

9.29 *cont'd*

Candidate	Mark in Anatomy	Mark in Physiology
A	60	70
B	29	60
C	51	60
D	53	35
E	45	50

9.30 Complete this table for the ranks from the last frame.

Candidate	Mark in Anatomy	Mark in Physiology
A	1	—
B	5	$2\frac{1}{2}$
C	3	$2\frac{1}{2}$
D	—	—
E	—	4
	Total = 15	Total = 15

1	1
5	$2\frac{1}{2}$
3	$2\frac{1}{2}$
2	5
4	4

9.31 When two candidates have the same score, what happens to their ranking? (B and C in Physiology in the last frame.)

They each get the arithmetical average of the rankings they would have taken if there had been a slight difference between them. This keeps the totals in the ranking columns the same. E.g. if there is a joint top, both rank $1\frac{1}{2}$, the average of 1st and 2nd. This principle extends to the case where more than two candidates have the same score.

9.32 Had E got 60 instead of 50 for Physiology in Frame 9.29 what would her/his rank have been?

B, C and E would, had there been a slight difference, have been 2nd, 3rd and 4th. As it is, they now all rank the *average*

$$= \frac{2 + 3 + 4}{3} = \text{3rd or 3.}$$

The sum of the ranks still equals 15. Notice that after these joint 3rd's comes the 5th.

9.33 d is the difference between a candidate's two rankings.
n is the number of pairs of results (candidates).
Use the formula for ρ given in Frame 9.27 to complete the calculation for the 2nd M.B. results in Frame 9.30.

As an arithmetical check you should find that because both ranks sum to the same totals, $\Sigma(d)$ always equals zero.

Candidate	Mark in Anatomy	Mark in Physiology	d	d^2
A	1	1	0	(ii)
B	5	$2\frac{1}{2}$	$2\frac{1}{2}$	$6\frac{1}{4}$
C	3	$2\frac{1}{2}$	(i)	(iii)
D	2	5	-3	9
E	4	4	0	0
	$\Sigma = 15$	$\Sigma = 15$	$\Sigma(d) = 0$	$\Sigma(d^2) = $ (iv)

(i) $= \frac{1}{2}$
(ii) $= 0$
(iii) $= \frac{1}{4}$
(iv) $= \Sigma(d^2) = 15\frac{1}{2}$

$n = ?$

$$\rho = 1 - \frac{6\Sigma(d^2)}{n(n^2 - 1)}$$

$= 1 - ?$

$=$

$n = 5$

$$\rho = 1 - \frac{6 \times 15\frac{1}{2}}{5 \times 24}$$

$= 1 - 0.775$

$= +0.225$

9.34 ρ is usually used (a) if the variables cannot be assumed to be normally distributed or (b) if no real score can be assigned but orders of preference can be given. For example, two surgeons discuss the various operations for gallstones. They are unable to give an actual numerical value for the relative efficiency for the operations so they .... them and calculate ....

rank
ρ

9.35   The results are on the opposite page. What is the value of ρ?

9.35	*cont'd*				

Operation	1st Surgeon's rank	2nd Surgeon's rank	d	d^2
A	1	3		
B	2	4		
C	3	2		
D	4	1		
	Total = 10	Total = 10	$\Sigma(d)$	$\Sigma(d^2)$

$n =$

$\rho =$

Now, $n = 4$

and $\Sigma(d^2) = 18$.

(Notice as a check that $\Sigma(d)$ always $= 0$.)

$$\therefore \rho = 1 - \frac{6 \times 18}{4 \times 15}$$

$$= -0.8$$

9.36　A third surgeon thinks operation B is the best and that the three others have equal merit. What rank values would he/she give the operations?

$A =$　$B =$　$C =$　$D = ?$

(Check that the rank total is the same as for the other surgeons.)

A = 3
B = 1
C = 3
D = 3

9.37　The range of ρ is the same as that for r.

The maximum value of ρ is ....

With no correlation ρ is ....

Like r, ρ has a .... and a .... value.

+1

0

sign, numerical

9.38　.......... is not so accurate as .... for measuring correlation as it does not take into account the actual results obtained (if these are available).

ρ, r
ρ is used when ranks are the only measures available or when the results are not normally distributed.

9.39　ρ is the rank order correlation coefficient described by .... and r is the product-moment correlation coefficient described by ....

Spearman

Pearson

9.40　Which correlation coefficient is easier to calculate?

Spearman's

9.41 To calculate these correlation
coefficients you need .... variables
measured on a group of .... people or
other subjects. When *r* is used, both
variables must be distributed ....; in
this case it is the more accurate
measure as the results themselves are
used. Sometimes it is only possible to
state a preference, or the data cannot be
assumed to be normally distributed, in
which case .... is calculated.

two

n

normally

ρ

9.42 Correlation coefficients of 1 never occur
in practice in biology or medicine. One of
the nearest is said to be that between
live weight and warm dressed weight of
poultry, where *r* = +0.98.

Incidentally, the scatter diagram below
represents *r* equal to +0.6, which will
help to give you some idea of the
correlation coefficient size.

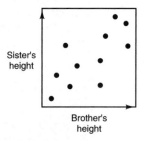

Sister's
height

Brother's
height

9.43 **Practical example**
x signifies erythrocyte sedimentation
rate;
y signifies the number of leucocytes in
thousands.
Both may be thought to be distributed
approximately normally.

Using the following results:

(1) Draw a scatter diagram.
(2) Guess the value of the correlation
    coefficient from the scatter diagram.
(3) Calculate *r*.
(4) Calculate ρ.

9.43 *cont'd*

x	y
1	3
2	5
3	5
5	2
5	4
5	6
7	7
7	10
9	8
10	12

(1) Scatter diagram

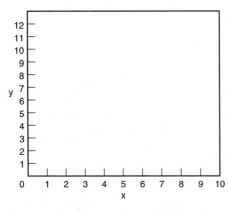

See page 253.

(2) Your estimate of the correlation coefficient =

(3) Calculation of r:

x	y	x^2	y^2	xy
1	3			
2	5			
3	5			
5	2			
5	4			
5	6			
7	7			
7	10			
9	8			
10	12			
$\Sigma x =$	$\Sigma y =$	$\Sigma(x^2) =$	$\Sigma(y^2) =$	$\Sigma(xy) =$

9.43 *cont'd*
$n =$

$$r = \frac{\Sigma(xy) - \dfrac{(\Sigma x)\,(\Sigma y)}{n}}{\sqrt{\Sigma(x^2) - \dfrac{(\Sigma x)^2}{n}} \ \sqrt{\Sigma(y^2) - \dfrac{(\Sigma y)^2}{n}}}$$

$=$

(4) Calculation of ρ

x	y	Ranked x	Ranked y	d	d^2
1	3				
2	5				
3	5				
5	2				
5	4				
5	6				
7	7				
7	10				
9	8				
10	12				
					$\Sigma(d^2)$

(Check that both ranks sum to 55 and $\Sigma(d) = 0$.)

$n =$

$$\rho = 1 - \frac{6\Sigma(d^2)}{n(n^2 - 1)}$$

$=$

$=$

Does r approximately equal ρ?

See page 254.

SUMMARY

The two most frequently used correlation coefficients are Pearson's and Spearman's.

Pearson's correlation coefficient is used when both variables are normally distributed. It is symbolised by r where

Summary *cont'd*

$$r = \frac{\Sigma(xy) - \frac{(\Sigma x)\,(\Sigma y)}{n}}{\sqrt{\Sigma(x^2) - \frac{(\Sigma x)^2}{n}}\ \sqrt{\Sigma(y^2) - \frac{(\Sigma y)^2}{n}}}$$

(n is the number of pairs of results).

Spearman's correlation coefficient is used when either of the two variables is not normally distributed, as well as when only ranks are available. It is not such an accurate measure as Pearson's in cases where Pearson's r would be appropriate; it is symbolised by ρ (rho) where

$$\rho = 1 - \frac{6\Sigma(d^2)}{n(n^2 - 1)}$$

and d is the difference between rankings.

Both r and ρ range from $+1$ to -1. They have sign and magnitude. $+1$ signifies maximum positive correlation, -1 means maximum negative correlation, and 0 means no correlation at all.

10. **Populations and samples**

INTRODUCTION

If you read some of the early volumes of the *Journal of the Royal Statistical Society* we think you would be surprised. In the 1830s research workers aimed to investigate entire populations; their task was usually impossibly hard and their work suffered accordingly. Today's research workers would consider only part – a sample – of each population and would draw their inferences from this. As you may imagine, these sample-to-population transplants are at best hazardous, with a lot of potential pitfalls. In medicine it is not enough to describe a patient: you have to assess the underlying condition. In statistics it is not enough to describe the results in the sample, you have to be able to assess the worth of the particular sample.

10.1   A population is an entire group about which some specific information is required or recorded. What is the population in Frame 1.9?

> All doctors in the newly developed African country.

10.2   The population is of prime importance as it is the subject of an experiment. It must be fully defined so that those to be included and excluded are clearly stated. For example, in the last frame you would need to know whether those doctors are included who are retired, part-time, or on leave, or who have in fact left that country while remaining on the register. Do you?

> No.
>
> 'All doctors' in that country is not a fully defined population without further specification.

10.3   In the population 'your medical faculty' you would include which of the following?

1) Teaching staff excluding part-time.
2) Teaching staff including part-time.
3) The medical librarian.
4) The medical students.
5) The cleaners in the medical school.
6) The bodies in the dissecting room.

> It is up to you. We would include 1) but this is not a very broad definition of the population. 'Your medical faculty' is not a fully defined population until we are all perfectly clear whom to include.

10.4	A statistical population need not be made up of people. We can have populations of birth weights, haemoglobin levels or blood cells so long as the population is what?	Fully defined
10.5	A *sample* is any part of the fully defined population. A syringe-full of your blood taken now is a sample of what population?	All your blood in circulation at the moment.
10.6	Sometimes, as above, a sample is the only means we have of inferring anything about a population. Sampling is also slower/quicker and cheaper/dearer than the complete enumeration of the population.	quicker, cheaper
10.7	Any inferences from a sample refer only to the particular population defined. Among a sample of patients in your teaching hospital it is found that only patients with cancer of the lung smoke more than 40 cigarettes daily. Does this indicate that smoking more than 40 cigarettes daily is associated with cancer of the lung?	Yes – pedantically, among the patients in your teaching hospital only.
10.8	Of course, this finding is nevertheless interesting, but only as a pointer to further research. The data on doctors in the newly developed African country tell you .... about doctors in neighbouring countries.	nothing
10.9	What is a sample?	Part of a defined population
10.10	What are $\bar{x}$ and s^2 the symbols for?	Mean and variance
10.11	In fact $\bar{x}$ and s^2 are the symbols for the mean and variance of the sample. Guess what μ and σ^2 are the symbols for.	The mean and variance of the population

10.12	μ and σ^2 are called mu and sigma squared. σ is pronounced .... and represents what?	Sigma. Standard deviation of the population.
10.13	σ is small sigma. Capital sigma is drawn .... and means	Σ, add together
10.14	A parameter is a constant used in describing a population. σ and μ are examples of parameters and $\bar{x}$ and s are examples of statistics. What is the difference between parameters and statistics?	Parameters refer to the population and statistics to samples from the population. Statistics are simply quantities defined in terms of the observations in a sample – in other words a function of those observations. However, note that we use sample statistics to estimate population parameters.
10.15	Statistics/parameters are used to infer about statistics/parameters.	statistics parameters
10.16	Each population has one/many value(s) of μ and one/many value(s) of σ.	one one
10.17	This is the frequency distribution of what?	A population

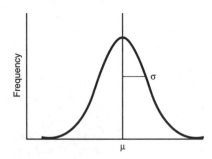

10.18	If you had not enumerated a population you could estimate σ by calculating s using which formula?	$s = \sqrt{\dfrac{\Sigma(x - \bar{x})^2}{n - 1}}$ or $\sqrt{\dfrac{\Sigma(x^2) - \dfrac{(\Sigma x)^2}{n}}{n - 1}}$

10.19 Statistics refer to samples. Parameters refer to populations. How can you remember this?

S and S
P and P

10.20 The size of the sample to be used is ideally a statistical consideration but is often limited in terms of t --- and c ---.

Time and cost
Often a compromise has to be reached between the various considerations. Sometimes the decision is reached that because it is just too costly (in terms of time and/or money) to take a sample that has acceptable statistical proportions, the sample will not be taken at all. This sort of consideration typically arises at the start of a clinical trial, for example, when deciding how many people are required in the trial.

10.21 For each population there is one value for every parameter, but for each population there are many possible samples each with their own .... estimating this parameter, i.e. for every μ there are many possible .... as estimates of it.

statistics

values of $\bar{x}$
Each value of $\bar{x}$ may differ slightly but they all should approximate to μ.

10.22 For every μ there are many possible $\bar{x}$'s taking aim and firing at μ!

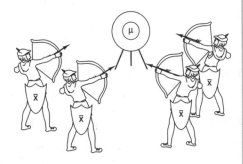

(a)

10.22   *cont'd*

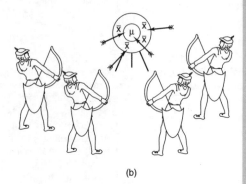

(b)

10.23   Good samples produce reliable ....
         while bad samples do not.

statistics
That is, good samples
produce reliable estimators
of the population
parameters.

10.24   The statistics shown in (a) are/are not
         better than those in (b).

are not
They are not such close
estimates.
Therefore in practice we
must design our methods
for choosing samples so
that, as in (b), we could
rely fairly well on any
possible value of $\bar{x}$.

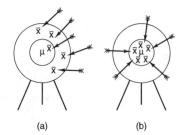

(a)   (b)

10.25   *Precision* is a term which indicates *how
         close* statistics (or estimates of a
         population parameter) *are* to *each other*.

10.26   *Bias* is the term which refers to *how far*
         the average statistic (or estimate of a
         population parameter) lies *from the
         parameter*.

10.27   Both these ideas are important and we
         should aim for precise, unbiased sample
         estimates, if possible.

It is not always possible to
achieve both these
objectives together, in
which case a compromise
becomes necessary.

10.28 In Frame 10.24 (a)/(b) is more precise and (a)/(b) is more biased.	(b) (the statistics lie closer together) (a) (the average statistic lies further from the parameter)

10.29 Here (a)/(b) is more precise but more biased.

(a) The statistics lie close together but are not close to the centre of the target.

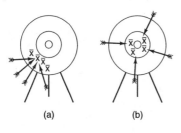

(a)   (b)

10.30 Good samples have statistics which are .... and ....

precise, unbiased

10.31 We will discuss bias again in the next chapter. We will conclude this chapter by talking further about precise statistics. What is precision?

How closely the statistics lie to *each other*

10.32 Remember that precision says nothing about whether statistics are on-target. However, an experiment which leads to estimates which are unbiased but without precision may still easily cause a statistic to be an off-target estimate. Below is a diagrammatic representation of such an experiment. If your particular estimate is .... it would not be very worthwhile.

$\bar{x}_1$ or $\bar{x}_6$

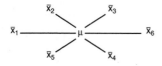

10.33 A measure of the precision of the sample mean, $\bar{x}$, from a random sample, can be defined as

$$\frac{\sqrt{n}}{\sigma}.$$

(This is intuitively reasonable – the smaller the variability, the greater the precision, and the greater the sample size, the greater the precision.)

Here n is the size of the sample and σ is ....

the standard deviation of the population

10.34 For any particular set of circumstances σ in the above formula is a constant. To vary precision, as defined by the formula, ... must be varied.

n or $\sqrt{n}$

10.35 To increase precision n must be decreased/increased.

increased
This is what you would expect – the bigger the sample the more precise the estimate.

10.36 From a sample of size 100, $\bar{x}$ is .... as precise as the mean from a sample of size 25.

Twice, since $\dfrac{\sqrt{100}}{\sigma}$ is twice as big as $\dfrac{\sqrt{25}}{\sigma}$.

10.37 To double the precision n must be ....

quadrupled (multiplied by 4)

10.38 Research workers often ask a statistician how large a sample they need to use. The reply depends on the level of precision required and the value of ....

σ

10.39 If you know how precise an estimate you need but do not know σ you can use a pilot survey to obtain an estimate of σ. You would in fact calculate .... from the pilot survey sample and substitute it in the formula:

s

10.39 *cont'd*
Estimated precision = $\dfrac{\sqrt{n}}{s}$.

Or you could use historical data from similar experiments in the past to estimate σ.

10.40 What is a sample?

Part of a defined population

10.41 From any particular sample you can estimate what?

The parameters – in the relevant, fully defined population only

10.42 Give two characteristics of a good statistic.

It is precise and unbiased.

10.43 What is precision?

How closely the statistics lie together

10.44 Precision of $\bar{x}$ from a random sample is estimated using what formula?

$\dfrac{\sqrt{n}}{s}$

10.45 n represents what?

The sample size

10.46 To increase precision what must you do?

Take a bigger sample

10.47 A sample which is too small may produce an $\bar{x}$ which is unbiased but which is too .... to draw valid conclusions.

imprecise

SUMMARY

It is not enough for you to be able to describe numbers – you must also be able to evaluate their worth when samples are used.

The population is the entire group in which you are interested. A sample is a portion of that population. The population must be clearly and exhaustively defined before a sample is drawn from it. If we are not sure whether a certain type of patient is included in the population because the population is not fully defined, we cannot be sure that any conclusion based on the sample refers to that particular type of patient. Any

Summary *cont'd*

conclusions based on information from the sample only refer to the particular population as defined. μ (mu) and σ (sigma) are parameters and refer to the population. $\bar{x}$ and s (respectively) are the equivalent statistics in the sample and are used to estimate the parameters. The only accurate way of estimating parameters is a complete population enumeration. Sampling is cheaper and quicker and is occasionally the only method of estimation available. The inference about a parameter using statistics is always hazardous, even with good samples.

One of the characteristics of a good sample is precise estimation, or, in the case of the mean, having the statistics $\bar{x}$ lying close together. Precision of the mean $\bar{x}$ can be measured by

$$\frac{\sqrt{n}}{\sigma}$$

where n is the sample size and σ the standard deviation of the population.

If σ is not known it can be estimated from a pilot survey or from historical data. To increase precision the sample size must be increased. For example, to double precision the sample size must be increased fourfold.

11. Fairness in sampling: how to be on-target

INTRODUCTION

We should aim for statistics to be both unbiased and precise.

11.1 .... is the term describing the closeness of statistics to each other.

Precision

11.2 What is bias?

The term describing how far the average statistic is from the parameter

11.3

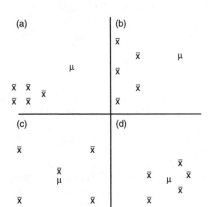

Above,

.... shows good precision but is biased;

(a)

.... shows good precision and is unbiased;

(d)

.... shows poor precision but is unbiased;

(c)

.... shows poor precision and is biased.

(b)

11.4 In the last frame .... represents the best state of affairs and .... represents the worst.

(d)
(b)

11.5	How do you improve precision?	Increase the sample size

11.6 Before we can minimise bias we must decide how it arises. Different sorts of bias, like different diseases, require different treatments.

If you wanted to find the average weight of adult males in a town you would/would not take as your sample the weights of the rugby team? Why?

would not
They would be a biased sample.

11.7 The commonest source of bias, as in the last frame, is the way in which the sample is selected. The treatment for bias in sampling is *randomisation*. One kind of random sample is the *simple random sample*, in which each member of the population has an equal chance of inclusion. If your population is not exhaustively and clearly defined can you have a *simple random sample*?

No. If you do not know the constitution of the population the members cannot have an equal chance of inclusion.
N.B. There are other kinds of random samples but we will not discuss them further in this programme.

11.8 A sample of 6 patients with disease X is required for a series of complicated tests from a population of 100 patients already numbered 00 to 99. Slips of paper numbered 00 to 99 are mixed well and the first 6 numbers drawn out are the sample. Is this a simple random sample?

Yes. All patients had an equal chance of being drawn; initially the members of the population were numbered consecutively and the required number of patients was drawn from the population.

11.9 Do the winning tickets in a lottery constitute a simple random sample?

Yes

11.10 What is a simple random sample?

One in which each member of the population has an equal chance of selection

11.11 What is an advantage of the simple random sample?

It guards against bias in selecting the sample.

11.12 To save time writing out numbers every time we want a random sample we can use instead published tables of random numbers, or we can generate random numbers from the computer. See page 278. These numbers were originally chosen so that they were free from bias. Instead of choosing 6 numbers between 00 and 99 we could read off 6 numbers each with 2 digits from the table of random numbers.
Look at the table of random numbers. Start at the top left–hand corner and read down the first 2 columns. Which are the 6 numbers which would constitute your random sample of patients?

Patients numbered
06
34
34
47
93
86
We will discuss the fate of patient no. 34, included twice, later. But in any case we will also read off the 7th number, namely 20, to allow us to have a sample of 6 different patients.

11.13 Remember that before drawing a random sample we must define the population and give each member a ....

number

11.14 If 660 patients had constituted the population we would need to read .... columns together rather than 2.

3

Otherwise those numbered in the hundreds could not be included.

11.15 If numbers turned up which were *bigger* than the number in the population we would ignore them and continue until we had filled the sample spaces with numbers of the required size. Why is it better to number a population of 100, 00 to 99 rather than 1 to 100?

In the latter case you would need to use 3 columns and would waste many of the numbers (since the 3 columns would only be required to account for one population member, namely number 100).

11.16 If the same number occurs twice in the table you would not include it twice in your sample, but you would reject it and choose another number from the table. From page 278, the 6th member of the sample in Frame 11.12 would then be patient number 20.
Can a person appear more than once in the sample?

No, not in practice. (Note that in theory, with sampling with replacement – i.e. you put back the one you have taken out each time you remove a member of the population – this can happen.) Patient 34 in Frame 11.12 would be rejected the second time.

11.17　It may be a source of bias in itself if you regularly use the tables and start at the same place (or if you look at the tables while deciding where to start). How can you avoid this?

Vary your starting point, deciding on it before seeing the tables. The starting point should also be decided randomly.

11.18　The numbers are read off consecutively from your selected starting point. The numbers can be read upwards, downwards or sideways. When is this decision taken?

Before seeing the tables Note that considerations of how to use the random number tables and thereby to produce a set of random numbers become unnecessary when we use computer-generated random numbers, which is the usual approach nowadays.

11.19　What is the variable in the table below?

Weight gained over a 2-month period for 100 one-year-old children.

Weight gained in gm by 100 one-year-old children in 2 months

Child's no.	Gain	Child's no.	Gain	Child's no.	Gain	Child's no.	Gain
00	879	25	936	50	1021	75	567
01	765	26	822	51	822	76	1049
02	652	27	907	52	849	77	765
03	936	28	1049	53	992	78	879
04	851	29	964	54	794	79	595
05	850	30	853	55	1162	80	936
06	1077	31	964	56	907	81	1021
07	936	32	794	57	852	82	879
08	709	33	822	58	822	83	1021
09	964	34	992	59	765	84	1049
10	737	35	936	60	907	85	1021
11	909	36	794	61	1077	86	964
12	624	37	539	62	964	87	709
13	794	38	907	63	624	88	848
14	482	39	1106	64	992	89	737
15	992	40	794	65	737	90	879
16	879	41	652	66	680	91	936
17	680	42	936	67	822	92	879
18	652	43	850	68	765	93	737
19	709	44	822	69	992	94	964
20	794	45	709	70	680	95	907
21	737	46	652	71	822	96	765
22	1134	47	624	72	765	97	879
23	936	48	1247	73	765	98	737
24	822	49	879	74	850	99	851

11.20	In the last frame the children are numbered 00 to 99, notice, rather than 01 to 100. How many columns do you need to read together to draw a random sample using the table of random numbers?	2

11.21   We want a random sample of 10 of these children. We have decided to start in columns 7 and 8, row 3 in the table of random numbers, reading sideways to the right first. What is the resulting sample of numbers? (See page 278.)

....

....

....

88	99	40	36
47	50	48	33
05	74		

36 is not included a second time, which is why 74, the 11th number from the table, is included.

11.22   Therefore, what is our sample of weight gains in gm using these random numbers to choose the 10 children from Frame 11.19?

....

....

....

848	851	794	794
624	1021	1247	822
850	850		

11.23   In our sample $\bar{x} = 870.1$ and $s = 163.6$ (compared with the population values $\mu = 851$ and $\sigma = 142$).
Do you think this is reasonably accurate?

It is, considering the sample is fairly small.

11.24   Now, guided by the scheme below, choose your own simple random sample of 10 children.

Column no.   =

Row no.   =

Direction   =

10 random numbers (from the table of random sampling numbers on page 278)
=

....

....

....

11.24   *cont'd*
10 weight gains in gm (Frame 11.19) =

....

....

....

Therefore your value of $\bar{x}$ =

and your value of s =

It is very unlikely that your own simple random sample will be identical to ours or anyone else's. All values of $\bar{x}$ and s should approximate to 851 and 142, though; do yours?

11.25   You may be thinking that the simple random sample is a lot of bother. You have a good point. Why is it used?

It is a sampling method which protects us from bias. In fact a simple random sample can occasionally produce off-target estimates but we can calculate the chances of this happening. It makes chance work for us rather than against us.

11.26   These are the steps in drawing a simple random sample by hand. Put them in order.

(a) Read off the sample of random numbers.

(b) Allot a number to each member of the population.

(c) Decide where to start in the table of random numbers.

(d) Refer the random sample of numbers to the population and read off the corresponding results.

(e) Decide in which direction to read the table of random numbers.

(b)

(c)

(e)

(a)

(d)

When a computer is being used to generate random numbers, this takes the place of steps (c), (e) and (a). Just as in (c) there is a procedure for choosing a random starting point.

11.27   The reason for the random sample is not so much that it necessarily leads to estimates which are unbiased but that it allows us to estimate the degree of bias we can expect. There is no short-cut to

No, even though people are trying to be fair it is surprising how bias creeps in when people use haphazard sampling methods.

11.27 *cont'd*
random sampling. Some people think *'haphazard'* samples are synonymous with random samples. To use this method you can go through the population and choose the ones which you feel like choosing. Is this an acceptable method?

11.28 Of what value is a 'haphazard' sample?

Very limited
No valid statistical inferences can be based upon such a sample since most statistical analytical procedures depend upon a random sample having been taken for their validity.

11.29 A random sample is often beyond the reach of many practising doctors. A biopsy specimen and a syringeful of blood are not random samples but they are nevertheless useful.
A particular doctor's patients are not a random sample of the local population from which they are drawn.
What should a doctor do if he discovers an interesting fact about them?
(1) Refuse to write it up in the journals because it is not a random sample.
(2) Write it up and call it a random sample.
(3) Write it up and point out it is a non-random sample.

(3) Then his work can be checked and followed up by others with more time or facilities.

11.30 If you read an article about an experiment in which no mention is made of whether it is in fact a random sample, what should you assume?

That it is not a random sample. If the author had gone to all the trouble of drawing a random sample he would have said so. Read the article with considerable caution.

11.31 Which is better – a non-random sample labelled as such or an undefined sample?

A non-random sample labelled as such. At least you know where you are.

11.32 Give two characteristics of a good sample.

It gives unbiased estimates to which a measure of precision may be attached.

11.33 Bias in sampling can be controlled. How?

By taking, for example, a simple random sample

11.34 What is a simple random sample?

One in which all members of the population are numbered and have an equal chance of selection

11.35 List the steps in taking a simple random sample.

Allot numbers.
Choose a starting point in the tables.
Choose the direction for reading the tables.
Read off the sample numbers.
Read off the results.
(Or use a computer to replace the steps using tables.)

11.36 Experiments almost invariably need a control sample as a yardstick against which to measure the evidence. A control group is one identical to the experimental sample in all respects except the factors under consideration. To serve this purpose the control sample needs to be selected ....

randomly

11.37 X-rays of adult males with a specified disease in a particular hospital are being investigated. What is the control group?

X-rays chosen at random of adult males without the disease in the same hospital. Sometimes in journals people omit a control group or use one which is in fact wrong in that particular experimental situation. If the experimental group is hospitalised it is wrong to compare it with people outside unless hospitalisation is the factor under review.

11.38 Even a properly controlled experiment can have biased results, especially if these results are *subjective* (based on opinion or what a person says) rather than *objective* (based on facts or what is measured). Are the following subjective or objective?

    (a) Haemoglobin levels
    (b) Patients' responses to a pain-killing drug
    (c) Birth weights
    (d) Number of cigarettes smoked daily

    (a) Objective
    (b) Subjective
    (c) Objective
    (d) The actual number is objective, but if the number is being estimated from memory it becomes subjective.

11.39 Subjective results can be very biased. Often a patient in a drug trial will sense what the doctor would like him to say. He might either deliberately try to please his doctor or displease him. Often a research doctor interprets subjective results subconsciously to fit in with his mood or theory. Does randomisation guard against this sort of bias?

No

11.40 These sources of bias tend to be limited by using 'blind' or 'double-blind' methods. A 'blind' experiment is one where the patient does not know in which group he or she is, for example, whether he or she is receiving the drug or not (the control group is often given an inactive tablet called a 'placebo'). A 'double-blind' experiment is one where neither the patient nor the doctor is aware of the treatment received by the patient. How does this improve the bias situation?

The patients in both the control and the other group will tend to be equally misleading. The doctor in the 'double-blind' situation cannot interpret the results to fit the particular theory.

11.41 How should a patient be allocated to a particular treatment?

At random

11.42 A psychiatrist wants to see whether a new drug called 'Snuze' is effective against insomnia. His results are to be in 'number of hours slept during the first week on the drug'.

11.42 *cont'd*

(1) How does he decide which patients receive 'Snuze'?

(1) At random among his patients suffering from insomnia.

(2) Which is the control group?

(2) Another group selected at random from his patients suffering from insomnia.

(3) The results are subjective/objective?

(3) Subjective, since the patients have to assess themselves how many hours they slept.

(4) The control group need/need not be given a placebo.

(4) The placebo is required.

11.43 Read this passage and then answer the following questions.

'An experiment is reported in a journal of physiology in which two different dietary regimes, A and B, were compared. Initially 120 normal and 25 under-weight children where chosen and weighed clothed. For a 6-month period the under-weight children were fed on dietary regime A and were given an antibiotic daily. The normal children were fed dietary regime B. At the end of the trial the mean weight gain of the under-weight children was greater than that of the normal children.'
The samples are/are not random?

They are not mentioned as being random, so presumably they are not.

11.44 The correct/incorrect control group has been used?

Incorrect. Both groups should either be normal or under-weight to begin with. Any difference in outcome could be due to this initial difference.

11.45 Why has the doctor given the antibiotic?

Even if this is ethical it is a further mistake as it adds another misleading factor. The difference could now also be due to the antibiotic.

11.46	It would/would not be better to weigh the children unclothed?	Would, because clothes vary in weight so children clothed vary more than when unclothed – so far as weight is concerned. When clothed, σ is bigger and therefore precision less.
11.47	The results are subjective/objective?	objective
11.48	He therefore need/need not use a blind experiment?	need not
11.49	From which sample is the mean, $\bar{x}$, more precise (assuming equal variances amongst the two types of children) and why?	The 120 normal children, because this sample is bigger.
11.50	Unfortunately, this sort of article has been published in the past. One further consideration is important when thinking about samples. This is whether the samples are chosen before embarking on the research *(prospectively)*, or whether patients already fall into the groups and it is only effects which are being compared *(retrospectively)*. Frame 11.43 is an example of a prospective/retrospective survey?	Prospective. The samples are chosen before the different diets were given.
11.51	A doctor has compared people who have had a heart attack with a control group to see whether their fat consumption has been higher. This is a prospective/retrospective study and what constitutes the control group?	Retrospective. The heart attack had already happened before the survey started. The heart attack patients were already grouped. The control group is a random sample of people identical save for the heart attack.
11.52	Retrospective studies are often so biased that they have been stigmatised as 'backward in two senses'. To make the experiment in the last frame a prospective study, you would do what?	Observe a group with a high fat consumption and a group with a low fat consumption and wait to contrast the rates of heart attacks.

11.53 Prospective studies are usually bigger. For example, if the average heart attack rate is 1 per 1,000 people, 100,000 would need to be observed prospectively to find 100 heart attack cases. Such studies are also usually more costly and time-consuming. What is their advantage?

They are usually less biased than their retrospective counterparts as the groups can be chosen randomly (and moreover facilities can usually be included at the same time to investigate other relevant factors).

11.54 If you compared the I.Q.'s of people with bilharzia with others is this a prospective or a retrospective study?

Retrospective. This shows another disadvantage with retrospective studies. If people with bilharzia were shown to be more stupid, you would be unable to say whether they had been stupid and contracted the disease or whether the disease had made them stupid.

11.55 What is the control group in the last frame?

The I.Q.'s of similar people without bilharzia.

11.56 Give two characteristics of a good sample.

It gives unbiased estimates on average, and their precision can be estimated.

11.57 The size of the sample affects the precision and/and not the bias.

and not

11.58 How can you guard against bias in sampling?

By using a random sample. At least it enables you to estimate the chance of bias creeping in.

11.59 In which of the following situations is bias a problem?

(a) Imprecise

(b) Objective

(c) Retrospective

(d) Non-random

(e) Subjective

(c), (d) and (e)
Retrospective
Non-random
Subjective

11.60   How do you guard against bias with a   Using a control (placebo)
         subjective experiment if you cannot   Using blind and double-
         make it objective?   blind experiments

11.61   **Practical example**
         A less knowledgeable colleague than   Some ideas are listed in
         you wants to compare two slimming   the Answers section on
         tablets. Tell him exactly what he must do   page 255.
         to produce satisfactory results.

SUMMARY

Bias produces unreliable results because the statistics consistently lie away from the parameter which they are to estimate – they are off-target.

Randomisation is the insurance against bias arising at the sampling stage. To choose a simple random sample the population members are numbered and tables of random numbers are used to read off the numbers of the population members to be included in the sample. The starting point and direction for reading the tables of random numbers are chosen before the tables are opened. Numbers occurring more than once are not usually in practice included in a sample more than once and higher numbers in the table than those used to number the population are ignored. Alternatively – and more likely nowadays – a computer can be used to generate a random sample.

Retrospective (backward-looking) studies are generally more biased than prospective studies although they are usually smaller, cheaper and quicker to perform.

Subjective results (based on opinion rather than facts) are more prone to bias then objective results. A control group (with a placebo in drug trials) and blind or double-blind experimental designs can be used to diminish the effect of bias with subjective results. The control group must be as like the group under investigation as possible except for the variable under consideration. It would also be chosen randomly.

The control group or contrast group is therefore a yardstick representing the norm against which the experimental group can be measured. If you read the medical literature with a critical eye you will probably find articles where an incorrect control group has been used.

Sometimes the wrong yardstick is used and sometimes no yardstick at all. As examples of wrong control groups we can find those which refer to another place, another time or season, or different age groups. People of different races are wrongly compared because the comparisons are not between those in the same income brackets, for example.

Dissimilarities in age, sex, social class, etc. can be brought into line by a method called standardisation. This is a procedure whereby one estimates what would have been the picture had the groups been balanced, e.g. for age.

Summary *cont'd*

Perhaps worst of all are the examples where no control groups are used at all. A disease situation is described in a particular group of people and we are left in the dark as to what is the normal picture in that place at that time for the general population of that age and sex. If there is no yardstick there can be no valid conclusion.

12. **What happens when we take samples**

INTRODUCTION

In the last chapter you calculated a value $\bar{x}$ to estimate μ for the weight gains. Samples taken by different people in this way are likely to have been different and $\bar{x}$ is likely, consequently, to have varied. The way $\bar{x}$ varies is important because usually you calculate only one value of a sample mean to estimate a population mean, and you want to know how reliable your estimate is likely to be. But your one value of the sample mean is just one of many possible values of the sample mean, which itself has a distribution – called the sampling distribution of the mean.

12.1	First, let us do a bit of revision. What is the difference between a parameter and a statistic, and what is a statistic?	A parameter refers to a population and a statistic to a sample. A statistic is simply some function of the sample data.
12.2	Now define 'a population'.	All of something under investigation
12.3	A sample is a .... of the population.	portion or part
12.4	How can you choose an unbiased sample?	Randomly
12.5	The statistic $\bar{x}$ estimates the parameter μ. How do you make $\bar{x}$ more precise?	Increase n, the size of the sample.
12.6	Do you remember what a 'variable' is? Why can $\bar{x}$ be called a variable?	Because it varies from sample to sample.
12.7	What is the approximate shape of the distribution of many variables?	Normal – bell-shaped, symmetrical with two points of inflection.
12.8	The distribution of $\bar{x}$ is no exception. Sketch the distribution of the sample mean.	

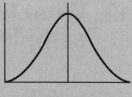

(If the samples are large.)

THE DISTRIBUTION OF THE SAMPLE MEAN

12.9 For the distribution, in fact, to be normal, the samples must be taken from a normal distribution and must be random.

This normal distribution of $\bar{x}$ when sampling from a normal distribution is another virtue of the random samples. (Note, however – and this is very important – that, if the samples are fairly large, $\bar{x}$ is distributed normally whether or not the underlying population distribution is itself normal. This is quite a remarkable result and an extremely useful one. When the population distribution is normal, this result holds even for small samples.)

12.10 What is an unbiased sample?

One where the *average* statistic is on-target or equals the parameter

12.11 Therefore, what is the average or mean value of the distribution of random sample means?

μ
If you got this answer right you can go straight to Frame 12.15. Otherwise go to the next frame.

12.12 Imagine a population from which lots of random samples have been taken (for example the population of 100 weight gains in the last chapter).

12.12 *cont'd*

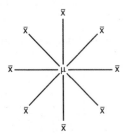

These values of $\bar{x}$ vary but are all nearly equal to ....

$\mu\ (= 851)$

12.13 In Frame 11.24 μ was 851, your value of $\bar{x}$ was .... and ours was 870.1.

Fill in your value $\bar{x}$ here:

12.14 Therefore mark your value of $\bar{x}$ here.

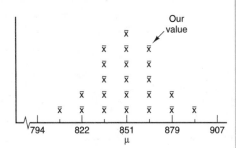

Values of $\bar{x}$

12.15 Draw the distribution of the sample mean, $\bar{x}$, as fully as possible.

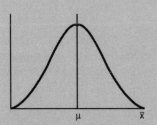

(The variable is usually shown at the far right end of the horizontal axis.)

12.16 What have you assumed in the last frame?

That the samples are random, and large

12.17 Once you know the value of the standard deviation you know all you need to know about the distribution of $\bar{x}$.

It is $\dfrac{\sigma}{\sqrt{n}}$.

You have met something like this already. What was it?

A measure of precision is

$$\frac{\sqrt{n}}{\sigma}.$$

So $\dfrac{\sigma}{\sqrt{n}}$ is $\dfrac{1}{\text{precision}}$.

If σ is not known, s can be used as its estimate.

12.18 This seems sensible. As the precision of $\bar{x}$ increases you would expect the variation of $\bar{x}$ to increase/diminish.

diminish

12.19 What is the variance of the distribution of $\bar{x}$?

$$\frac{\sigma^2}{n}$$

12.20 What does n represent?

The size of the sample

12.21 If n is multiplied by 4 (i.e. you quadruple the size of your sample), the standard deviation of the distribution of $\bar{x}$

$\left(\dfrac{\sigma}{\sqrt{n}}\right)$ is .... and the precision

halved

$\left(\dfrac{\sqrt{n}}{\sigma}\right)$ is ....

doubled

12.22 Sketch the distribution of $\bar{x}$ taken from large random samples.

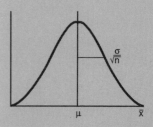

12.23 $\dfrac{\sigma}{\sqrt{n}}$ is so important it is given a special name and a special symbol.

$\dfrac{\sigma}{\sqrt{n}}$ = *the standard error of the mean* =

$\sigma_{\bar{x}}$ or $s_{\bar{x}}$ (= $\dfrac{s}{\sqrt{n}}$) if σ is not known

Write the formula for precision using this new symbol.

Precision = $\dfrac{1}{\sigma_{\bar{x}}}$ or $\dfrac{1}{s_{\bar{x}}}$ if σ is estimated by s.

12.24

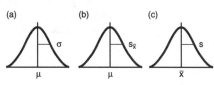

(a)　　　(b)　　　(c)

In the above, ... is the distribution of a population.

.... is the distribution of a sample from a population.

.... is the distribution of random sample means.

a

c

b

12.25 The value of σ for I.Q.'s of university students is 15. Suppose that you take a random sample of size 9. What is the value of $\sigma_{\bar{x}}$?

$\dfrac{15}{\sqrt{9}}$ = 5

12.26 What is $s_{\bar{x}}$ called?

The standard error of the mean. It is the sample estimate of $\sigma_{\bar{x}}$ when σ is unknown.

12.27 What value had $\sigma_{\bar{x}}$ for the distribution of sample means of weight gain in Frame 11.24?

$\dfrac{142}{\sqrt{10}}$ = 44.9

12.28 If you did not know σ how would you estimate $\sigma_{\bar{x}}$?

Use s instead of σ, to give

$\dfrac{s}{\sqrt{n}}.$

12.29 State a formula for calculating s.

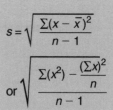

$$s = \sqrt{\frac{\Sigma(x - \bar{x})^2}{n - 1}}$$

$$\text{or} \sqrt{\frac{\Sigma(x^2) - \dfrac{(\Sigma x)^2}{n}}{n - 1}}$$

12.30 What are this distribution and its standard deviation called and what exactly does the distribution represent?

Distribution of the sample mean
Standard error of the mean
The distribution of all the means of large random samples of size n from a given population.

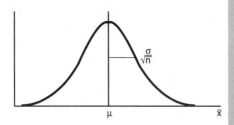

12.31 If you alter the size of your sample you do not change the value of the mean/standard deviation of the distribution of $\bar{x}$ but the mean/standard deviation of this distribution does change.

mean
standard deviation

12.32 A random sample has two virtues. What are they?

It is not unrepresentative of the population from which it was taken in any systematic way and the values of $\bar{x}$ follow a defined distribution, the distribution of the sample means.

12.33 Sketch the distribution mentioned in the last frame.

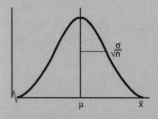

Often research workers wish to compare two means.

For example, soon we are going to see whether the mean birth weight of offspring of diabetic mothers differs significantly from that of normal mothers using the data from Chapter 3. Initially we assume that there is no difference between the means of the underlying populations from which the samples are taken. To understand this fully later we will now take a quick look at:

THE DISTRIBUTION OF THE DIFFERENCE BETWEEN TWO SAMPLE MEANS

12.34 From its name what do you think the variable is in the above-mentioned distribution?

$(\overline{x}_1 - \overline{x}_2)$, where the subscripts 1 and 2 refer to the two different samples

12.35 You can imagine how the variable $(\overline{x}_1 - \overline{x}_2)$ is distributed – how?

Normally

12.36 This is so, whatever the distributions of the populations, under what conditions?

If the samples are random and large

12.37 What was your value of $\overline{x}$ in Chapter 11, again .... ?

12.38 Ours was 870.1. What value does $(\overline{x}_1 - \overline{x}_2)$ have in this case?

(your value minus 870.1) or (870.1 minus your value), depending on which sample we label 1 and which we label 2.

12.39 Suppose that you constructed a number of samples and computed a value $\overline{x}$ for each sample, and that we did the same for the same number of samples. What distribution would the values of the form $(\overline{x}_1 - \overline{x}_2)$ follow, pairing off your samples and our samples, and subtracting the means?

The distribution of the difference between two sample means. (n is in fact small, but as σ is known the distribution is normal, as will be explained later.) The full distribution of the differences is called the sampling distribution of the difference between two sample means.

12.40 Most values of $\overline{x}$ are close to ...., which they estimate.

μ

12.41 Some are a little bit bigger and on average an equal number are a little bit smaller than μ. Therefore what do you think the *average* value of $(\bar{x}_1 - \bar{x}_2)$ equals?

0
Some answers are a little bit bigger and others a little bit smaller, but the average difference is 0.

12.42 Sketch the sampling distribution of the difference between two sample means, showing the variable $(\bar{x}_1 - \bar{x}_2)$ at the far right-hand side of the horizontal axis.

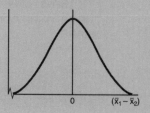

12.43 The standard deviation for the distribution of the mean, again, is what?

$$\frac{\sigma}{\sqrt{n}}$$

12.44 The variance in this distribution equals what?

$$\frac{\sigma^2}{n}$$

12.45 It is a fact that the variance of the distribution of the difference between two sample means is

$\frac{\sigma^2}{n_1} + \frac{\sigma^2}{n_2}$ where n_1 and n_1 are the sizes of the two samples.

This variance in words equals what?

Note that the population variance is the same for both samples here since we have arranged that the two samples are taken from the same population. More generally we will be interested in cases where the samples are taken from *different* populations – e.g. different treatment groups of patients.

The sum of the variances of the two individual sample means. This result sometimes surprises people. So let us repeat it. The variable of the *difference* between the sample means is the *sum* of the variances of the sample means.

12.46 That is, the variance of the distribution of $(\bar{x}_1 - \bar{x}_2)$ is $\frac{\sigma^2}{n_1} + \frac{\sigma^2}{n_2}$.

What is the standard deviation of this distribution?

$$\sqrt{\frac{\sigma^2}{n_1} + \frac{\sigma^2}{n_2}}$$

In case you are worried by this, there will be no more complicated algebra than this in this programme.

12.47 In our random samples from the weight gains in Frame 11.24 the values of n were equal to .... and σ = ...

10, 142
Note that in general the sample sizes might be different (n_1 and n_2, say).

12.48 The distribution of $(\bar{x}_1 - \bar{x}_2)$ for these weight gains had a variance
$$\frac{\sigma^2}{n_1} + \frac{\sigma^2}{n_2}$$
equal to what number?

$$\frac{142^2}{10} + \frac{142^2}{10} = 4033$$

12.49 The standard deviation
$$\sqrt{\frac{\sigma^2}{n_1} + \frac{\sigma^2}{n_2}}$$
equals what number?

63.5

12.50 Algebraically
$$\sqrt{\frac{\sigma^2}{n_1} + \frac{\sigma^2}{n_2}} = \sigma\sqrt{?}$$

$$\sqrt{\frac{\sigma^2}{n_1} + \frac{\sigma^2}{n_2}}$$
$$= \sqrt{\sigma^2\left[\frac{1}{n_1} + \frac{1}{n_2}\right]}$$
$$= \sigma\sqrt{\frac{1}{n_1} + \frac{1}{n_2}}$$
$$= \sigma\sqrt{\frac{n_1 + n_2}{n_1 n_2}}$$

12.51 Which distribution is this?

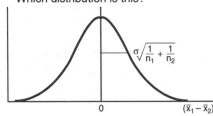

The distribution of the difference between two sample means

12.52 How big are the samples?

n_1 and n_2

12.53 What kind of samples are they?

Random

12.54 What distribution is this?

A population distribution

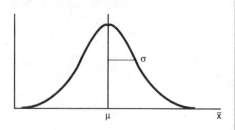

12.55 What distribution is this?

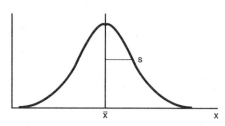

A sample distribution
Note that only in a large sample would the shape of the distribution approach the smooth curve shown here. $\bar{x}$ is an estimate of μ, and s is an estimate of σ, so the distribution then approximates the population distribution. For small samples the sample distribution will not be represented by a smooth curve, though $\bar{x}$ and s are still estimates of μ and σ, respectively.

12.56 Sketch the distribution of the sample mean, $\bar{x}$, when the samples are random and large.

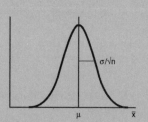

12.57 What is $\dfrac{\sigma}{\sqrt{n}}$ called and what is its symbol?

The standard error of the mean $\sigma_{\bar{x}}$, estimated by $s_{\bar{x}}$

12.58 What exactly is the distribution of the sample mean?

The distribution of all sample means of random samples of size n drawn from a population

12.59 Sketch the distribution of the difference between two sample means, $(\bar{x}_1 - \bar{x}_2)$.

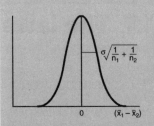

12.60 What exactly is this distribution?

The distribution of the difference between two sample means, one based on a random sample of size n_1 and one based on a random sample of size n_2.

SUMMARY

Frames 12.54 to 12.60 serve well as the summary. You need to recognise these distributions when we use them again later.

Most readers of the earlier editions found that this was the most difficult chapter in the whole book. The significance tests used in Chapters 16 and 17 to analyse actual research data are based on the two sampling distributions covered in this chapter. You will be able to perform these tests without fully understanding this chapter, but of course you will be performing them rather in the dark. Should you be unhappy about the contents of this chapter we suggest you read it again now before proceeding. It would be far better for you to be able to perform the tests covered in Chapters 16 and 17 *with* an understanding of what you are doing.

Note: sample means follow the normal distribution, at least approximately, if the samples are large and random, whatever the shape of the distribution in the population – and the larger the sample, the better the approximation. If the population distribution is normal, $\bar{x}$ also follows the normal distribution, even in small samples.

13. **The laws of chance**

INTRODUCTION

The last chapter was fairly difficult, compared with others in this programme, so well done for getting to this one! However, with this chapter and the following chapter, we have all the props for applying significance tests to results which are normally distributed. So it has been worth getting this far, to provide you with the statistical tools that you will need.

This chapter itself is the basis for *all* statistical tests.

13.1 Many people talk about the likelihood, chances or odds of a particular event happening. We use the word *probability*. What is the probability of tossing 'tails' with a fair coin? (Note: a probability is a number between 0 and 1.)

1/2, or 0.5

13.2 Probability is often given the symbol 'p'. Its range is 0 to 1. When $p = 0$ an event is impossible. What does $p = 1$ mean?

That an event is inevitable

13.3 What is p that you will die one day?

1, sadly

13.4 State an event for which $p = 0$.

Possible examples are: your swimming the Atlantic, or our winning the Booker prize for this book.

13.5 Sometimes p can be estimated logically. The probability of drawing an ace from a normal card pack is 1/13, i.e. you have 1 chance out of 13, since there are 4 aces out of 52 cards, and 4/52 = 1/13. Other times you can estimate p empirically from the equation:

$$p = \frac{\text{total number of occurrences of the event}}{\text{total number of trials}}$$

If a surgeon transplanted 200 hearts and one person survived for more than one year the probability of survival for more than one year here is what?

$\dfrac{1}{200}$

To be more precise, this is the estimate of the probability of a heart transplant patient, treated by that particular surgeon, surviving for more than one year.

13.6 This means *p* is equivalent in form to

$$\frac{\text{the number of sheep}}{\text{total number of animals}}$$

which is an example of a ....

proportion

13.7 The probability, *p*, equals .... that a fair coin will fall 'heads' and equals .... that a '2' will be thrown with one fair die.

$\frac{1}{2}$

$\frac{1}{6}$

13.8 If any one event precludes the possibility of other specified events, the events are called *mutually exclusive*. Surviving an operation, refusing an operation and succumbing during the operation are/are not mutually exclusive events.

They are. Each of the three possibilities excludes the other two. Falling into one of the groups excludes you from the others.

13.9 Tossing a head *or* a tail with one throw of a coin does/does not mean mutually exclusive events.

It does. If the word 'or' appears it infers mutually exclusive events.

13.10 Tossing a head with one coin *and* a tail with another coin are/are not mutually exclusive.

They are not – you can do both. Note the use of the word 'and' here, rather than 'or'.

13.11 So long as events are mutually exclusive the *Addition Law of Probability* states the following:
The probability that an event will occur in *one of several possible ways* is the sum of the individual probabilities of these separate events.
Therefore, what is the probability of throwing a '6' *or* a '2' with one particular die of a set of fair dice?

$\frac{1}{6} + \frac{1}{6} = \frac{1}{3}$

13.12 For the addition law to apply, the word '*or*' is seen or implied. Remember the events must be mutually exclusive. What is the probability of drawing an ace *or* a king with one cut from a pack of cards?

$\frac{1}{13} + \frac{1}{13} = \frac{2}{13}$

13.13 Is the probability of drawing an ace and a king with two cuts from the pack

$$\frac{2}{13}?$$

No – they are not mutually exclusive events. You have two draws and can do both. The addition law does not apply.

13.14 What is the probability of tossing a 'head' *or* a 'tail' with one throw of a fair coin?

$$\frac{1}{2} + \frac{1}{2} = 1$$

i.e., it is inevitable.

13.15 When all possible outcomes of mutually exclusive events are given, their probabilities sum to one. The probability of throwing a '3' with one die + the probabilities of throwing what? = 1.

Anything but a 3, i.e. a 1 or a 2 or a 4 or a 5 or a 6 with that throw

13.16 The probability of being blood group rhesus +ve equals 1 minus which probability?

The probability of not being rhesus +ve (i.e., rhesus -ve) – its corresponding mutually exclusive event

13.17 The probability of being rhesus -ve is $\frac{1}{10}$.

What is the probability of being rhesus +ve?

$$1 - \frac{1}{10} = \frac{9}{10},$$

because the events are mutually exclusive. (So the Addition Law of Probability can be used here to *subtract* one probability from 1 to calculate the desired answer.)

13.18 What are mutually exclusive events?

Those events for which the occurrence of one of the events precludes any of the other events from occurring

13.19 What does the Addition Law of Probability state?

That with mutually exclusive events, to find the probability of one or another (or others) happening, the individual probabilities are added

13.20 What is the sum of the probabilities of a group of all possible mutually exclusive events?

1

13.21 Suppose that the probability of a successful pregnancy resulting in a multiple birth is

$$\frac{1}{80}.$$

Amongst those pregnancies which result in at least one birth, what is the probability of a single birth?

$$1 - \frac{1}{80} = \frac{79}{80}$$

13.22 The addition law on its own is of limited use. The probability of a single birth is

$\frac{79}{80}$ and of being rhesus +ve is $\frac{9}{10}$.

We cannot use the addition law to determine the probability of a single rhesus +ve birth.
Why ?

Because these events can occur together. They are not mutually exclusive.

13.23 The *Multiplication Law of Probability* applies to two or more events which do not affect each other (i.e. are independent) occurring together. Does it apply to mutually exclusive events?

No, these cannot occur together

13.24 What are independent events?

Those which do not affect each other

13.25 Rhesus blood grouping and multiplicity of births are independent events. The probability of a rhesus +ve

birth is $\frac{9}{10}$ and that of a single birth is

$\frac{79}{80}$.

What, therefore, is the probability of a successful pregnancy resulting in a single rhesus +ve birth?

$$\frac{9}{10} \times \frac{79}{80} = \frac{711}{800}$$

(The multiplication law applied to independent events.)

13.26 If the probability of a female birth is $\dfrac{1}{2}$

what is the probability of a female rhesus +ve birth?
(These are also independent events.)

$$\dfrac{1}{2} \times \dfrac{9}{10} = \dfrac{9}{20}$$

13.27 The probability of a birth which is female, single and rhesus +ve equals ....
(*Hint*: the multiplication law extends to apply to more than two events.)

$$\dfrac{1}{2} \times \dfrac{79}{80} \times \dfrac{9}{10} = \dfrac{711}{1600}$$

13.28 If the events involved are associated (not independent of each other), the multiplication law cannot be applied. The probability of being colour–blind is

$\dfrac{1}{12}$ and of being female is $\dfrac{1}{2}$.

Is the probability of being born female

and colour-blind $\dfrac{1}{24}$?

No. Colour blindness is generally associated with sex; most colour-blind people are male – the multiplication law does not apply to two such associated events.

13.29 What is the probability of throwing a 6 *or* a 2 with a single throw of a fair die?

$$\dfrac{1}{6} + \dfrac{1}{6}$$

(Addition law again)

13.30 For the multiplication law to apply the word *'and'* is used to connect the events. For the addition law the word .... connects them.

'or'

13.31 What is the probability of throwing a 6 with the first throw of a fair die *and* a 2 with the next?

$$\dfrac{1}{6} \times \dfrac{1}{6} = \dfrac{1}{36}$$

(Multiplication law)

13.32 What is the probability of throwing a 2 first and then a 6 with a fair die?

$\dfrac{1}{36}$ – the same

13.33 Therefore what is the probability of throwing a 6 and then a 2 *or* a 2 and then a 6 (i.e. a 2 and a 6 either way).

$$\dfrac{1}{36} + \dfrac{1}{36} = \dfrac{1}{18}$$

13.33 *cont'd*

(Addition law, applied to the two probabilities obtained from the multiplication law.)

13.34 Consider the same ideas in the sex of two siblings. What is the probability of

(a) a male and then a male?

(a) $\dfrac{1}{4}$

(b) a male and then a female?

(b) $\dfrac{1}{4}$

(c) a female and then a male?

(c) $\dfrac{1}{4}$

(d) a female and then a female?

(d) $\dfrac{1}{4}$

(These are mutually exclusive and do in fact sum to 1.)

13.35 Therefore what is the probability of two siblings being one male and one female (in either sequence)?

$$\frac{1}{4} \quad + \quad \frac{1}{4} \quad = \quad \frac{1}{2}$$

male then   female then
female   male

(Again, this makes use of both the multiplication law and the addition law.)

13.36 Complete this table for two offspring:

Sequence	Family	Probability
M M	2 males	$\dfrac{1}{4}$
F M	1 male and	$\dfrac{1}{4}$ $\Big\}$ $= \dfrac{1}{2}$
M F	1 female	$\dfrac{1}{4}$
F F	2 females	?

$\dfrac{1}{4}$

13.37   Notice that the probability of one female and one male is twice that for two males. This is because two males can only arise in one sequence but one of each sex can arise in .... sequences.

two
If events can occur in more than one sequence the overall probability is the sum of the probabilities for each sequence.

13.38   7 males in a family only arise in one sequence: male and male and male etc. What is the probability of 7 offspring all being male?

$$\frac{1}{2} \times \frac{1}{2} \times \frac{1}{2} \times \frac{1}{2} \times \frac{1}{2}$$
$$\times \frac{1}{2} \times \frac{1}{2} = \left(\frac{1}{2}\right)^7 = \frac{1}{128}$$

13.39   6 males and 1 female can arise in .... sequences:

7

i.e.   M M M M M M F or
        M M M M M F M or
        M M M M F M M or
        M M M F M M M or
        M M F M M M M or
        M F M M M M M or
        F M M M M M M

Each of them has a probability $\left(\frac{1}{2}\right)^7$ so that the overall probability is what?

$$\left(\frac{1}{2}\right)^7 + \left(\frac{1}{2}\right)^7 + \left(\frac{1}{2}\right)^7 + \text{etc.}$$
$$= 7 \times \left(\frac{1}{2}\right)^7 = \frac{7}{128}$$

13.40   The number of sequences in which 2 females can arise is 21. The probability for 2 females and 5 males in

any order is $\frac{21}{128}$.

Similarly the probability of 3 females = $\frac{35}{128}$ and so on.

These probabilities are represented in the diagram.

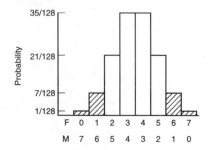

13.40 *cont'd*
All these alternatives are mutually exclusive.

What is the total probability?

1

13.41 Probability can be represented by size of area so long as the total possible area equals .... and the area is drawn to scale.

1

13.42 What is the probability of 7 children consisting of 0 or 1 females *or* 0 or 1 males?

(Corresponds to the shaded area in Frame 13.40.)

$$\frac{1}{128} + \frac{7}{128} + \frac{7}{128}$$

$$+ \frac{1}{128} = \frac{16}{128} = \frac{1}{8}$$

This is the same as the probability of 1 or no patients preferring drug A in a drug trial, or of 1 or no patients preferring drug B, where the probability of preferring one drug or the other is $\frac{1}{2}$ and where 7 patients try each of two drugs, A and B. (Separately of course!)

13.43

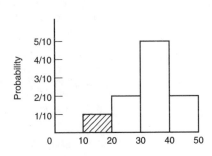

What is the probability of having a value less than 20 in this histogram? (It is the shaded area.)

$$\frac{1}{10}$$

(The area is 1/10 of the whole.)

13.44 What is the probability of a result greater than μ in this population distribution?

$$\frac{1}{2}$$

13.44   *cont'd*

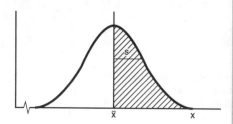

13.45   What does probability mean?

The chance of a particular outcome relative to all the possible outcomes.

13.46   If the chances are 50 : 50, the corresponding probability, *p*, = ...

$\dfrac{1}{2}$

13.47   Give the formula for estimating *p* empirically.

$$\dfrac{\text{Total number of occurrences}}{\text{Total number of trials}}$$

13.48   When would you add probabilities together?

With mutually exclusive events when wanting the probability of one event *or* another (or others).

13.49   When would you multiply probabilities?

When the probability of two or more events occurring together is required (so, connected by the word '*and*') and they are not associated.

13.50   When events can occur in more than one sequence the overall probability is the ....

sum of the probabilities for the individual sequences

SUMMARY

Probability means the chance of an event occurring, relative to all the possible outcomes. It often has the symbol '*p*' and ranges from 0

Summary *cont'd*
(impossibility) to 1 (inevitability). It is estimated empirically from the formula:

$$\frac{\text{total number of occurrences of the event}}{\text{total number of trials}}$$

The *Addition Law of Probability* applies to mutually exclusive events which are events such that the occurrence of any one event excludes the possibility of any other taking place. The probability of one *or* more mutually exclusive events is the sum of the individual probabilities. All the probabilities of mutually exclusive events sum to one.

When the word *'and'* replaces *'or'* we use the *Multiplication Law of Probability* such that the probability of two or more events occurring together is the product of their individual probabilities. This is only true if the events are not associated in any way, i.e. if they are independent.

When events can occur in more than one sequence the overall probability is the sum of the probabilities for the individual sequences.

Where the total area is one unit, proportional area can be used to represent probability.

14. Standardising the normal curve

INTRODUCTION

In this chapter we learn to apply the ideas about probability to the normal distribution. This is the last stage before going on to use numbers to answer questions.

14.1 What is the frequency distribution which many variables follow approximately in medicine?

The normal distribution

14.2 You are about to learn about a new characteristic feature of the normal curve. What characteristics do you already know?

It is symmetrical and bell-shaped with two points of inflection.

14.3 The new characteristic concerns probability, denoted by p. Is probability a ratio, a proportion or a rate?

A proportion
Probability can be expressed as:

$$\frac{\text{Number of occurrences of an event}}{\text{Total number of trials}}$$

14.4 A percentage is 100 times a ratio/rate/proportion?

proportion

14.5 What is the *percentage* area beyond $(\mu + \sigma)$ here?

16%

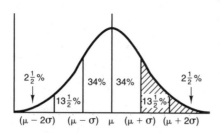

$2\frac{1}{2}\%$ 34% 34% $2\frac{1}{2}\%$

$13\frac{1}{2}\%$ $13\frac{1}{2}\%$

$(\mu - 2\sigma)$ $(\mu - \sigma)$ μ $(\mu + \sigma)$ $(\mu + 2\sigma)$

14.6 What is the proportion of area beyond $(\mu + \sigma)$ in the last frame?

0.16

14.7	Therefore, what is the *probability* of a result being bigger than $(\mu + \sigma)$ in that normal curve?

0.16

14.8 These probabilities and percentage areas apply to all normal curves. What is the probability of obtaining a result lower than two standard deviations below the mean (*i.e.* below $(\mu - 2\sigma)$ in Frame 14.5)?

$p = 0.025$ ($2\frac{1}{2}\%$)
It is the same as that above $(\mu + 2\sigma)$.

14.9 Here is a curve representing the distribution of I.Q.'s in some population. What is the probability of having an I.Q. above 130? (Refer to Frame 14.5 if you need to and assume for the purpose of answering this question that I.Q. is a continuous variable – this is not strictly true, but the answer will be a good approximation to the true result.)

$130 = (\mu + 2\sigma)$. The probability equals that above $(\mu + 2\sigma)$, i.e. $p = 0.025$.

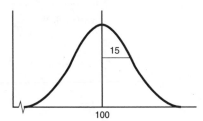

14.10 This curve represents the distribution of haemoglobin levels in some population. What is the probability of having a haemoglobin level above 110?

0.025, the same as in Frame 14.9

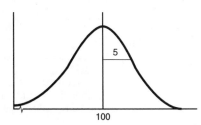

14.11 You are as unlikely to have an I.Q. of 130 or bigger as to have a haemoglobin level of 110 or above. Why is this?

Because both the values 130 and 110 lie 2 standard deviations beyond the mean on a normal curve.

14.12 Here the probability beyond $7\frac{1}{2}$ on Graph B is the same as beyond .... on Graph A.

1

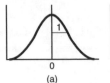 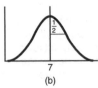

(a)   (b)

14.13 On Graph (a) in the last frame the value 2 lies .... standard deviation(s) above the mean, and -1 lies .... standard deviation(s) below the mean.

2
1

14.14 In fact in Graph (a) in Frame 14.12 the numerical value itself tells you the number of standard deviations you are from the mean.
-3 on this normal curve is where?

3 standard deviations below the mean

14.15 Because Graph (a) in Frame 14.12 has special features it is given a special name – the *standard normal curve*. The special features are as follows:
It has a mean value ....
It has a standard deviation .... and variance ....
Not only is this particular normal distribution easy to work with, but it is the *only* one that is tabulated – and it is the only one that needs to be tabulated.

0
1
1

14.16 Below is a drawing of the standard normal curve. The variable is given the symbol .... and represents what?

Z. (*z* is a particular value of *Z*.)
The number of standard deviations from the mean on a normal curve.

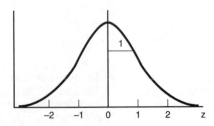

14.17 What is the probability of a *z* value less than −1 on the standard normal curve? (The diagram from Frame 14.5 is repeated here after modification.)

0.16

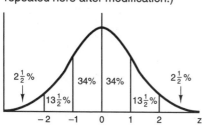

14.18 A *z* value of −1 on the standard normal curve corresponds to the value (............) on all normal curves.

$\mu - \sigma$

14.19 Conversely the result $8^{1}/_{2}$ on normal curve B in Frame 14.12 is equivalent to .... on the standard normal curve.

$+3$
It is 3 standard deviations above the mean.

14.20 To recap, the *z* value on the standard normal curve equals ....
....
....
on all normal curves.

the number of standard deviations above or below the mean

14.21 With the result 70 here, *z* = ...

−2

14.22 By calculating *z* as in the last frame every value on any normal curve can be related to the .... normal curve. This is why the standard normal curve is the only one that needs to be tabulated.

standard

14.23 The z value equals the number of standard deviations from the .... on any normal curve.

mean

This equals

$$\frac{\text{the distance from the mean}}{\text{the standard deviation}}$$

i.e. $z = \dfrac{\text{the particular result} - \text{the mean}}{?}$

the standard deviation

14.24 Using this formula, the value 4 on the normal curve with mean 10 and standard deviation 6 is equivalent to a z value of what?

$$\frac{4 - 10}{6} = -1$$

14.25 This means it lies .... standard deviation(s) .... the mean.

1
below

14.26 Therefore the probability of obtaining a result equal to or lower than 4 on a normal curve with mean 10 and standard deviation 6 is what?

0.16

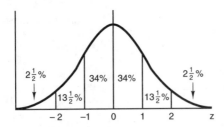

14.27 Give the formula for calculating z.

$z =$

$z = \dfrac{\text{the result} - \text{the mean}}{\text{the standard deviation}}$

14.28 The formula for z in the last frame can/cannot be used for all normal distributions.

It can. This is the purpose behind the standard normal curve and z.

14.29 This diagram relates z to ....

the probability p, of obtaining a higher or lower value of z.

14.29 *cont'd*

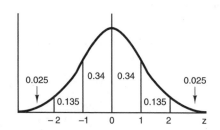

14.30 Therefore any value on any normal curve can be related to .... by first calculating ....

p
z

14.31 Very often, in using the normal curve to answer questions, we are interested, at the same time, in values bigger than $+z$ or smaller than $-z$.
In Frame 14.29 the probability *p* of a result bigger than $z = +2$ or smaller than $z = -2$ is ....

We are interested in both tails in what are called 'two-tailed tests'.

0.05
(0.025 + 0.025)
(Note that this is an approximate result. The exact values of *z* corresponding to this probability are $z = +1.96$ and $z = -1.96$.)

14.32 Instead of using the standard normal curve itself we can construct tables of *z* and the equivalent *p* values. Using the diagram in Frame 14.29 and the result from the last frame we have

p: 0.32   ?

z: 1   2

? = 0.05

14.33 Do you understand where the 0.32 came from in the last frame where $z = 1$?

Yes, we hope so. 16% of results are beyond $z = +1$ and 16% below $z = -1$ giving a total of 32%, i.e. $p = 0.32$.
(The *z* value and *p* value refer to both ends of the normal curve together.)

14.34 Useful values for z (N.B. plus or minus) and the equivalent p values are given below:

p	0.10	0.05	0.02	0.01
z	1.64	1.96	2.33	2.57

Explain again what $z = 1.96$, $p = 0.05$ means.

The probability of a result bigger than $z = +1.96$ or smaller than $z = -1.96$ is 0.05.
Of course, 1.96 is very close to 2. So it follows that the total probability in the two tails of the standard normal distribution, beyond 2 standard deviations from the mean, is approximately 0.05.

14.35 z is the variable on which curve?

The standard normal curve

14.36 z represents ....
....
and may be calculated using the formula $z = ?$

the number of standard deviations from the mean

$$z = \frac{\text{the result} - \text{the mean}}{\text{the standard deviation}}$$

14.37 Use it, and the table for Frame 14.34 (which has been transferred to page 274 at the back of the book) to answer the following question.
What is the probability of a result bigger than 22.9 or smaller than 9.1 in a normal distribution of mean 16 and standard deviation 3?

$$z = \frac{22.9 - 16}{3} \text{ or } \frac{9.1 - 16}{3}$$

$= +2.3$ or -2.3
From the table, p is 0.02.

14.38 In the table, p includes both ends of the curve. If you had only been interested in the last frame in the probability of a result bigger than 22.9 you would have .... the p value given in the table.

halved
Note that in using statistical tables generally, it is very important to know exactly what is being tabulated. This should be defined in the tables, often with diagrams to help you.

14.39 Complete the diagram below to indicate from the table $z = 2.3$ where $p = 0.02$.

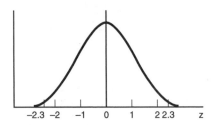

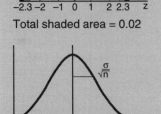

Total shaded area = 0.02

14.40 Sketch the distribution of the sample mean! (From memory, we hope.)

14.41 For any particular result $\bar{x}$ from this normal curve,

$z =$
(using the formula)

$\dfrac{\text{the result} - \text{the mean}}{\text{the standard deviation}}$

$= \dfrac{\bar{x} - \mu}{\dfrac{\sigma}{\sqrt{n}}}$

Use this in the next frame.

14.42 Assume that psychology students have an average I.Q. of 120 with a standard deviation 15. You perform I.Q. tests on a random sample of 36 such students and calculate $\bar{x}$ to be 125. What is z's value and the probability of such an $\bar{x}$ value as 125 or bigger turning up?

$\bar{x} =$

$\mu =$

$\sigma =$

$n =$

$z =$

$p =$ (from the tables)

but, $p =$ (here)

$\bar{x} = 125$

$\mu = 120$

$\sigma = 15$

$n = 36$

$z = \dfrac{125 - 120}{\dfrac{15}{\sqrt{36}}} = +2$

The equivalent value of p is approximately 0.05 from

14.42 *cont'd*

the tables. We only want the 'or bigger' end and therefore the required probability is approximately 0.05/2 = 0.025.

14.43 95% of the results lie between .... and .... here.

$(\mu + 1.96\sigma)$
$(\mu - 1.96\sigma)$
(or, approximately,
$(\mu + 2\sigma), (\mu - 2\sigma))$

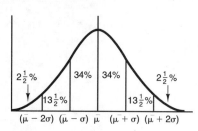

14.44 Look at the distribution of the sample mean below and compare it with the last frame.

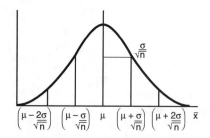

95% of sample means lie between .... and ....

$\left[\mu + \dfrac{1.96\sigma}{\sqrt{n}}\right]$ and $\left[\mu - \dfrac{1.96\sigma}{\sqrt{n}}\right]$

(or, approximately,

$\left[\mu + \dfrac{2\sigma}{\sqrt{n}}\right]$ and $\left[\mu - \dfrac{2\sigma}{\sqrt{n}}\right]$)

14.45 We can be 95% certain that a value of $\overline{x}$ is within .... of μ.

$\dfrac{1.96\sigma}{\sqrt{n}}$

$\left(\text{or approximately, } \dfrac{2\sigma}{\sqrt{n}}\right)$

14.46 Sometimes μ is unknown and we require to estimate it using $\bar{x}$. We are 95% confident that our particular $\bar{x}$ is within .... of μ.

$$\frac{1.96\sigma}{\sqrt{n}}$$

14.47 $$\left[\bar{x} - \frac{1.96\sigma}{\sqrt{n}}\right] \text{ and } \left[\bar{x} + \frac{1.96\sigma}{\sqrt{n}}\right]$$

are called the 95% *confidence limits* for estimating μ. If σ is unknown the 95% confidence limits for μ may be written .... and ....

These confidence limits provide a range of possible values for μ that are consistent with the data. They have been calculated so that for 95% of all such random samples limits calculated in this way will capture the true value of μ, but over the remaining 5% of samples they will not!

We are 95% confident that μ lies within the interval between

$$\left[\bar{x} - \frac{1.96s}{\sqrt{n}}\right] \text{ and } \left[\bar{x} + \frac{1.96s}{\sqrt{n}}\right]$$

i.e. approximately $\left[\bar{x} - \frac{2s}{\sqrt{n}}\right]$

and $\left[\bar{x} + \frac{2s}{\sqrt{n}}\right]$

This is provided, of course, that the sample is random and also that the sample is fairly large.

14.48 We wish to estimate μ for the I.Q. of all university students. We take a random sample of 100 students and find the mean result in this sample to be 115 with standard deviation 10. We are 95% confident that μ is between

$$\bar{x} - \frac{1.96s}{\sqrt{n}} \text{ and } \bar{x} + \frac{1.96s}{\sqrt{n}},$$

or, approximately, $\bar{x} - \frac{2s}{\sqrt{n}}$

and $\bar{x} + \frac{2s}{\sqrt{n}}$

which equals .... and .... here.

$$115 - \frac{2 \times 10}{\sqrt{100}} \text{ and}$$

$$115 + \frac{2 \times 10}{\sqrt{100}}$$

$= 113$ and 117

14.49 The distribution of the sample mean is normal only if the samples are ....

random and fairly large or the underlying distribution is normal.

14.50 The 95% confidence limits expressed in the above form can only be used to estimate the position of μ if the sample is .... and ....

random, fairly large
(Say more than 30 if σ is unknown.)

14.51 .... and .... are the ends of the 95% confidence interval for μ if the sample is random.

$$\left[\bar{x} - \frac{1.96\sigma}{\sqrt{n}}\right] \text{ and } \left[\bar{x} + \frac{1.96\sigma}{\sqrt{n}}\right],$$

or, approximately,

$$\left[\bar{x} - \frac{2\sigma}{\sqrt{n}}\right] \text{ and } \left[\bar{x} + \frac{2\sigma}{\sqrt{n}}\right]$$

14.52 When is such a 95% confidence interval used?

When we need to estimate a parameter (e.g. μ) from a statistic ($\bar{x}$) and we are interested in variation in both directions (two tails).

14.53 We calculate the mean birth-weight of a random sample of 36 children of diabetic mothers to be 3119 g with a standard deviation of 851 g. What can we say about the mean birth-weight of all such babies?

We are 95% confident it lies between

$$3119 - \frac{1.96 \times 851}{\sqrt{36}} \text{ and}$$

$$3119 + \frac{1.96 \times 851}{\sqrt{36}}$$

$$= 2841 \text{ g and } 3397 \text{ g}$$

14.54 Complete again the distribution of the difference of two sample means.

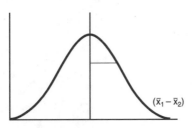

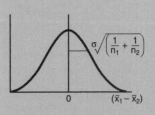

14.55 You have a particular value of $(\bar{x}_1 - \bar{x}_2)$.

Which formula would you use to calculate the equivalent value of z?

$$z = \frac{\text{the result} - \text{the mean}}{\text{the standard deviation}}$$

$$= \frac{(\bar{x}_1 - \bar{x}_2) - 0}{\sigma\sqrt{\left[\frac{1}{n_1} + \frac{1}{n_2}\right]}}$$

$$= \frac{\bar{x}_1 - \bar{x}_2}{\sigma\sqrt{\left[\frac{1}{n_1} + \frac{1}{n_2}\right]}}$$

14.56 $z = \dfrac{\bar{x} - \mu}{\dfrac{\sigma}{\sqrt{n}}}$ and $z = \dfrac{\bar{x}_1 - \bar{x}_2}{\sigma \sqrt{\left(\dfrac{1}{n_1} + \dfrac{1}{n_2}\right)}}$

will be used again soon.
You do not need to remember them,
though we hope you could derive them
for yourself. Could you?

Yes, we hope so.

14.57 Sketch the standard normal curve.

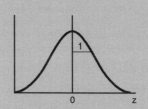

14.58 z = the number of what?

Standard deviations from
the mean

14.59 What is the importance of the standard
normal curve?

The z value can be
derived for all results from
normal curves.

14.60 Using what formula for z?

$z = \dfrac{\text{the result} - \text{the mean}}{\text{the standard deviation}}$

14.61 Sketch the value of p used in tables
relating p to z, where z equals 1.64.

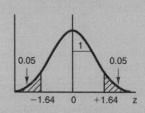

14.62 If you are interested in only one end of
the curve how can you use the table?

Use half the recorded
value of p.
This is the situation in
what are called 'one-tailed
tests', which you will learn
about soon.

SUMMARY

All normal curves can be adjusted so that the probability of obtaining certain results or bigger can be calculated. They can be adjusted to the standard normal curve which has mean equal to 0 and standard deviation 1. The result of the standard normal curve, z, equals the number of standard deviations that a result on any other normal curve lies from the mean. z can be calculated using the formula:

$$z = \frac{\text{the result} - \text{the mean}}{\text{the standard deviation}}.$$

Therefore, for the distribution of the sample mean

$$z = \frac{\bar{x} - \mu}{\dfrac{\sigma}{\sqrt{n}}},$$

and for the distribution of the differences between two sample means

$$z = \frac{\bar{x}_1 - \bar{x}_2}{\sigma\sqrt{\left[\dfrac{1}{n_1} + \dfrac{1}{n_2}\right]}}.$$

Tables relating p to z are readily available. In the table given here, the tabulated p value is the probabilities of obtaining a result bigger than $+z$ or less than $-z$ added together. To obtain the probability at one end of the curve from this table the tabulated p value is halved. When you use other statistical tables this might be different. You need to inspect the tables carefully to see what is being tabulated.

A confidence interval can be used to predict a likely range of values for a parameter in a population using statistics from a sample. The most commonly used confidence limits are used to predict the value of μ from $\bar{x}$. The 95% limits when σ is also unknown are, in large random samples,

$$\left[\bar{x} - \frac{1.96s}{\sqrt{n}}\right] \text{ and } \left[\bar{x} + \frac{1.96s}{\sqrt{n}}\right], \text{ i.e. approximately } \left[\bar{x} - \frac{2s}{\sqrt{n}}\right] \text{ and } \left[\bar{x} + \frac{2s}{\sqrt{n}}\right].$$

By substituting results from a random sample in these formulae we have an interval within which we are 95% confident that μ falls, on condition that the sample is fairly large (say bigger than 30).

Let us return for a moment to the consideration of the normal distribution of some variable, rather than of the mean of a sample. Often in medicine we are concerned with normal ranges of laboratory values for some variables. Now, because 5% of normal results fall outside the central 95% of the distribution, an isolated pathological test result on a patient which is beyond the normal limits as quoted by the pathologist does not necessarily make that patient's result abnormal. On the contrary, it is to be expected that a proportion of fit people will have what we might term 'sick results'. Similarly, of course, normal results (i.e. within the expected normal limits) can arise in people whose diseases would cause one to anticipate results beyond the norm.

Summary *cont'd*

Pathological results must be assessed in conjunction with the mathematical yardsticks proffered by the pathologists. While this is true, normals and abnormals fall on both sides of these values and so the rest of the clinical picture is also important.

Well done for getting to this point! From now on we will largely be able to use the ideas that we have already met.

15. Ideas behind significance tests

First, a short story, which is partly true.

A physician and a surgeon traditionally went to play golf on Thursday afternoons (time and weather permitting). At the nineteenth hole it was decided that they should each toss a coin. Should both toss 'heads' or both toss 'tails' they would re-toss their coins until the unfortunate one threw a 'head' (and bought the drinks) and the other one threw a very profitable 'tail'. On the first three occasions the physician tossed 'tails' and the surgeon 'heads'. The surgeon bought the beverages very willingly. On the fourth successive occasion the surgeon emptied his pocket rather less willingly.

Returning home after the fifth successive Thursday's expenditure, the surgeon muttered to his wife: 'I'm sure *the physician is above board*, but I do think there is something rather uncanny in his "tail-tossing" ability'. However, the surgeon's wife was able to reassure her husband: 'It is obviously just bad luck on your part *due entirely to chance* – ignore it.' The sixth week the surgeon tossed the unlucky 'head' yet again. Although feeling rather anti-physicians, he did not comment. After the seventh game the surgeon's wife was faced with a very belligerent husband. She agreed that enough was enough. Even though there was no proof that the physician was employing a trick (for these results could be entirely due to chance) it was very suspicious. *'The line must be drawn somewhere'*, she said. 'If it happens again, you must play golf with somebody else.'

Ideas like these are very commonly used in analysing experimental data, although the circumstances are usually rather different. The story has some statistical morals.

1. Any set of results involving data subject to chance variation, could be *'due entirely to chance'* as the surgeon's wife pointed out. Statistics can never *prove* anything.
2. Statisticians initially assume that chance is the only factor. Like the surgeon, they give the benefit of the doubt – they assume *'the physician is above board'*. The surgeon's wife initially thought that the results were *'due entirely to chance'*, too.
3. In statistical significance tests, as in the story, the time comes when *'the line must be drawn somewhere'*. Otherwise, no conclusions can be drawn – no action taken. Chance could always be to blame, but the time comes when the evidence is such that it is more realistic to assume some other factor.

INTRODUCTION

In earlier times medical progress, when it occurred, tended to leap forward, e.g. the discovery of the use of B_{12} and insulin. The results were obvious. However, in the last few decades many advances have been made by a series of research workers, each contributing a small improvement to the overall picture. On such occasions the only way to decide that an improvement really exists is by careful experimental design and analysis.

In this chapter we consider the ideas behind the general format of all significance tests.

15.1 Scientific research usually follows these steps:
   a) *observation* of a phenomenon,
   b) *postulation* of a theory to account for the observation,
   c) *prediction* of a result on the basis of the theory,
   d) *experiment* designed to test the prediction,
   e) *analysis* of the experimental results,
   f) *conclusion* as to whether or not to accept the theory.

   With which of these steps is statistics involved?

   d, e and f

15.2 Sometimes people say that the very nature of medical data particularly, with their inherent variability, makes their scientific analysis impracticable. This is rubbish – statistics depends on variability for its very existence. If all patients reacted in the same way we could use simple arithmetic. However, statistics can only supply a measure of doubt, not ....

   proof

15.3 As the surgeon's wife in our story said, the results could always be what?

   Due entirely to chance

15.4 Statistically, like the surgeon's wife, we always initially assume that the results obtained are *'due entirely to chance'* variation. This is the same as the legal approach, a kind of initial guilt/innocence.

   innocence

15.5	The idea in italics in the last frame is called the Null Hypothesis in statistical jargon. Look at Frame 11.43 again. What was the Null Hypothesis? Note that the Null Hypothesis is often *not* the one that we believe in.	That any difference between these regimes, as indicated by the results, was only due to chance
15.6	The *alternative* to the Null Hypothesis is that the results obtained indicate that there is a situation which is more than we can reasonably account for by chance. What is the Null Hypothesis?	That the results are only due to chance
15.7	*'The line must be drawn somewhere.'* Persistently saying that the Null Hypothesis could always be true, gets us nowhere. The time must come when the evidence is such that we must stop supporting the Null Hypothesis and give our allegiance to the	alternative
15.8	When this point is reached our conclusion is that we now accept/reject the Null Hypothesis and accept/reject the alternative theory.	reject accept
15.9	Dr D is conducting a drug trial to decide whether a particular type of pneumonia responds better to injections of: a) long-acting penicillin, b) crystalline penicillin. What is the Null Hypothesis and its alternative?	The Null Hypothesis is that any difference is just due to chance variation. The alternative is that the difference in response is more than can be expected by chance.
15.10	Initially we assume the Null Hypothesis is true. Does the value A, here, support the Null Hypothesis more than the value B?	Yes. It is nearer the centre where no difference is specified.

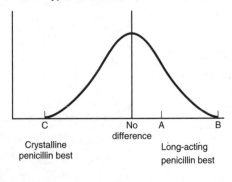

15.11 In the last frame B could still be due to chance variation (the Null Hypothesis) but it is more likely due to ....

the alternative that there is a real difference

15.12 In Frame 15.10:

With result A we would .... the Null Hypothesis.

accept

With result B we would .... the Null Hypothesis.

reject

With result C we would .... the Null Hypothesis.

reject

15.13 With result D here would you:
a) reject the Null Hypothesis?
b) accept the Null Hypothesis?
c) not know what to do?

You say:
a) You are easily convinced.
b) You are a doubting Thomas.
c) You must make up your mind.

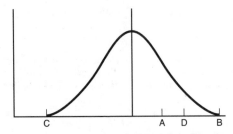

15.14 We must make up our minds and draw some conclusion with the point D. As the surgeon's wife said in the story, 'The line must be drawn somewhere'. The actual line is called the *significance level*. We usually reject the Null Hypothesis with extreme results at either end of the scale. Therefore we need a significance level at both ends.

What conclusion may be reached about D now?

With result D and this significance level we still accept the Null Hypothesis.

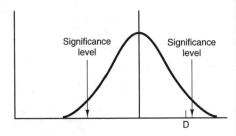

15.15 Why is a significance level necessary?

It enables decisions to be made.

15.16 You could choose any significance level you like but one commonly used, the 0.05 level shown below, is such that the *total* probability of a more extreme result at *either* end is 0.05.
The shaded area under this curve represents how much of the total?

The total shaded area is 0.05 or 5%, as the 0.05 significance level includes the probability at either end.

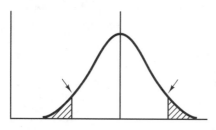

15.17 What does the 0.05 significance level (often referred to as the 5% significance level) mean in the case where 100 trials are performed?

That, on average, in 5 of these trials a more extreme result would occur by chance

15.18 The other commonly chosen level is called the .... significance level shown below.

0.01 (or 1%)
(0.005 at each end)
Occasionally the 0.001 level is used.

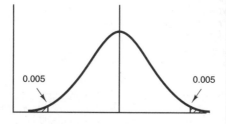

0.005   0.005

15.19 The .... is the yardstick against which the evidence in support of or against the Null Hypothesis is measured.

significance level

15.20 What is the 0.05 significance level?

The line at which the probability of a more extreme result is 0.05

15.21 Imagine the Null Hypothesis is on trial. Initially we, the jury, believe him innocent but there is some possibility of being wrong. The probability of us being correct to support him is called p. If p is more than the significance level we accept/reject the Null Hypothesis.

accept
There is insufficient evidence yet to cause us to disbelieve the Null Hypothesis.

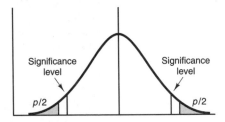

Note: In the diagram p is smaller than the significance level.

15.22 The value p is the probability of such a result or a more extreme result than the one obtained, arising by chance. The smaller p, the less the evidence to support the Null Hypothesis and the greater the evidence to support the

....

Alternative Hypothesis

15.23 The recent trend has been towards quoting the actual significance level achieved from a particular experiment – the p value – rather than simply declaring a result significant or not at some prespecified level. This is more informative for the reader who is then presented with the full weight of evidence from the data. After all, p values of 0.049 and 0.051 are very close together, yet if we were working strictly at the 5% significance level, the outcomes would be quite different – rejection of the Null Hypothesis in the first case, acceptance of the Null Hypothesis in the second case.

15.24 If p is less than 0.01 it is more/less significant than if it was only less than 0.05.

more

15.25 This symbol > means 'is bigger than'. At the end of an article in a journal you read '0.05 > p > 0.01'. Therefore what conclusion is drawn at the 0.05 significance level?

0.05 is bigger than p. Therefore p is less than 0.05. The Null Hypothesis is rejected and you accept the real difference alternative. Note that more recently, you have been likely to see a statement such as $p = 0.032$ in the article – this is more informative.

15.26 '0.05 > p > 0.01' At the 0.01 significance level your conclusion would be ....

that you still accept the Null Hypothesis The evidence has not yet crept beyond this significance level.

15.27 You read '0.01 > p' (or, perhaps more likely, 'p < 0.01'). What is your conclusion?

You reject the Null Hypothesis and accept the alternative at this significance level.

15.28 If you calculate p to be 0.04, relative to the 0.05 level, 0.05 .... p (symbol) and your conclusion is?

$0.05 > p$ You reject the Null Hypothesis and accept the alternative theory.

15.29 These are the steps in performing a significance test. Number them in the correct order.
a) Calculate p.
b) State the Null Hypothesis and its alternative.
c) Draw conclusions.

a) is 2nd

b) is 1st

c) is 3rd

15.30 Dr C wonders whether more boys or more girls get a particular complication of bilharzia. The population is all children suffering from bilharzia. Of the 7 cases reported 6 were male and 1 female. *(Fictitious Data)* State the Null Hypothesis and its alternative.

The Null Hypothesis is that any difference between boys and girls in the incidence of the complication is due to chance. The alternative is that there is a real difference between boys and girls with regard to the complication of bilharzia.

15.31 Initially we assume the Null Hypothesis is correct. Therefore, the probability of a boy suffering the complication rather than a girl by chance is ...., assuming that equal numbers of boys and girls suffer from bilharzia.

$\frac{1}{2}$

15.32 Look at Frame 13.40 again. What is the probability of the 7 cases being 6 boys and 1 girl?

$\frac{7}{128}$

15.33 The p value is the probability of such a result or a more extreme result occurring by chance (including both ends of the scale). From Frame 13.40 p equals .... (the shaded areas)

$p =$
$\frac{1}{128} + \frac{7}{128} + \frac{7}{128} + \frac{1}{128} = \frac{16}{128} = 0.125$

(7 of one sex is more extreme than 6 to 1, and both ends are included.)

15.34 $p = 0.125$
Your conclusion?
(Your p value is greater than the significance levels.)

You accept the Null Hypothesis at all significance levels because $p > 0.05$ and $p > 0.01$.

15.35 You have just performed your first significance test. List the stages.

a) State the Null Hypothesis and Alternative Hypothesis.
b) Calculate p.
c) Draw the conclusion.

15.36 Assume all 7 cases had been males. By completing the 3 stages, perform the significance test again.
a) The Null Hypothesis and alternative remain the same.
b) Your p value (Frame 13.40) is
    ....
c) Your conclusion is ....

$p = \frac{1}{128} + \frac{1}{128}$
$= 0.016$
$0.05 > p > 0.01$

p is less than 0.05 – you accept the alternative at this level.

p is more than 0.01 – here you still accept the Null Hypothesis.

15.37   The different significance levels have resulted in a different conclusion. Less evidence is required to accept an alternative theory at the 0.05 significance level (5% significance level) than at the 0.01 significance level (1% significance level). This is the reason why a theory accepted at the 0.01 significance level (1% significance level) is said to be more 'significant'. It is also the reason why if you accept the Null Hypothesis it can be due to one of two causes.

Either: there is insufficient evidence as yet to accept the alternative

or

....

there is in fact no real difference

15.38   To distinguish between these two causes you must do what to your samples?

Increase their size

15.39   Occasions arise when the theory does not involve both ends of the scale, but only one. A new drug may be more expensive and, unless it is better than the old one, people are not interested. They are not interested in which outcome?

Whether the old drug is better than the new one

15.40   When only one end is important the significance levels used are still 0.05 and 0.01, but the probability areas now only apply to one end, i.e. for the one-tailed test here the shaded area is .... of the whole area.

0.05 or 5%

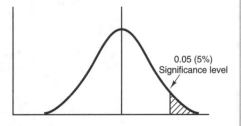

0.05 (5%)
Significance level

15.41	When the significance level only refers to one tail, of course, the p value you calculate also only applies to that tail. If $p > 0.05$, your conclusion, as before, is	that you accept the Null Hypothesis – either there is no real difference or there is insufficient evidence.
15.42	Another time when only one tail is used is when previous knowledge can exclude one possible extreme. Mrs H's theory is that bilharzia lowered the I.Q. of the patient (she knows it does not increase it). The stated .... enables you to decide whether both or only one tail should be used.	alternative to the Null Hypothesis
15.43	Frame 11.43 required one/both tail(s). Why?	Both. The theory relates to either of the dietary regimes being better. With one end we would only be interested in one regime being better.
15.44	A drug company runs an early phase trial of a new drug, Y, and its older counterpart, X, on a small group of patients, to see whether Y is better than X. Six patients responded better to Y and one to X. (Each patient received each drug but with a sufficiently long time interval in between so that there was no carry-over of the effect of the drug.) This requires use of one/both tail(s).	One. We are only concerned with the new drug being better than the old.
15.45	To draw conclusions from the last frame we must follow what steps?	a) State the Null Hypothesis and alternative. b) Calculate p. c) Draw conclusions.
15.46	State the Null Hypothesis and its alternative.	That any difference is due to chance. (Null) That Y is better than X. (Alternative)
15.47	What is the probability of a patient improving more with drug Y than drug X, assuming the Null Hypothesis is correct?	$\dfrac{1}{2}$

15.48	To calculate p here you do/do not include both ends.	do not
15.49	Using Frame 13.40 again, p here =	$$\frac{1}{128} + \frac{7}{128} = \frac{8}{128}$$ $$= 0.06$$ Remember p is the probability of the result or a more extreme result occurring by chance, but only at one end here.
15.50	Symbolise this result using the significance level, p, and the 'greater than' sign ($>$).	$p > 0.05$
15.51	Therefore what conclusion do you draw?	Either there is no difference or there is insufficient evidence to indicate that drug Y is better than drug X.
15.52	To distinguish between these two conclusions in the last frame you must do what?	Increase the sample size
15.53	What is the first stage in performing a significance test?	State the Null Hypothesis and its alternative
15.54	What decision is based on this alternative?	Whether one or both ends of the scale are to be used
15.55	What does the Null Hypothesis state?	That any difference is due to chance
15.56	What is the purpose of a significance level?	It enables decisions to be made
15.57	Which significance levels are commonly used?	0.05 (5%) and 0.01 (1%) (occasionally 0.001 (0.1%))

15.58 A significance level of .... enables more alternatives to the Null Hypothesis to be accepted. However, with it the Null Hypothesis will be wrongly rejected in .... cases out of 100.

0.05 (5%)

5, on average. (This is a price you must pay to reach a conclusion.)

15.59 Your next step in performing a significance test is to calculate p. What does p represent?

The probability of such an extreme or more extreme result occurring by chance, assuming the Null Hypothesis is correct.

15.60 If p is less than the significance level, what is your conclusion? (e.g. $p < 0.01$.)

The Null Hypothesis is rejected and the alternative accepted.

15.61 Otherwise, if $p > 0.05$, what is your conclusion?

Either there is insufficient evidence to reject the Null Hypothesis or there is no real difference.

15.62 **Practical example**
Look back at the golfing story, where the surgeon was left puzzling about the physician's ability to toss 'tails' so consistently. After how many rounds should the surgeon's wife have persuaded her husband to call a halt?
Remember, if they both tossed heads or both tossed tails they threw again. Ignore the probability of this happening and just calculate, the Null Hypothesis being assumed correct, the probability of the surgeon throwing heads and the physician tails and vice versa for an increasing number of times until the significance levels are passed.
Notice this probability is the same as that of patients stating a preference for one of two drugs in a cross-over trial (i.e. where the patients cross over from taking one drug to taking the other). Answer is on page 255.

SUMMARY

Statistics deals with material subject to inherent variability and helps by providing a measure of doubt about theories. These theories can never be proved. Significance tests enable research workers to draw conclusions.

The stages in performing a significance test are:

a) State the Null Hypothesis and its alternative.
b) Calculate p.
c) Draw conclusions.

The Null Hypothesis states that the experimental results are not due to the theory, but only due to chance variation. It is accepted as true until sufficient evidence is collected to reject it.

The usual significance levels are 0.05 (5%) and 0.01 (1%). They are the yardsticks against which the evidence is measured. The 0.05 (5%) significance level means that in 5 times out of 100 (a probability of 0.05) such an extreme value or a more extreme value would occur by chance. This is the price the experimenter is prepared to pay in adopting this significance level. Rejecting the Null Hypothesis at this level means that 5 times out of 100, or 1 in 20 times on average, the experimenter would be making the wrong decision (rejecting the Null Hypothesis when, in fact, it is true). This is what is called a Type I error. The Null Hypothesis is rejected more often if the 0.05 (5%) level is used rather than the 0.01 (1%) level and more significant differences are found. The failure to reject the Null Hypothesis when it is in fact wrong is a Type II error. If we can be wrong all the time with significance tests you may doubt their value. Their value is only that they give us a measure for our doubts about the reality of observed differences and they facilitate decisions being made.

Two examples of conclusions:

A. Two-tailed test, 0.05 (5%) significance level

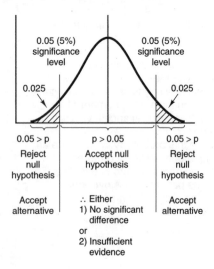

Summary *cont'd*
B. One-tailed test, 0.01 (1%) significance level

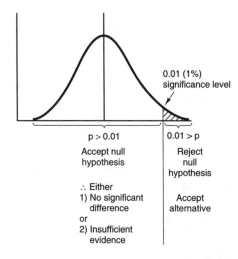

The *p* value for the experimental result is the probability of the actual experimental result or more extreme results arising by chance alone. Usually *p* includes the equally extreme results at both ends of the scale (a two-tailed test). In this case the significance levels also include both ends. If one end of the scale can be excluded on theoretical grounds, the *p* value and significance levels only apply to the relevant end (a one-tailed test).

If $0.05 > p > 0.01$ the alternative is accepted at the 0.05 (5%) significance level, but not at the 0.01 (1%) level. An alternative to the Null Hypothesis accepted at the 0.01 (1%) level is more 'significant' than one at the 0.05 (5%) level. Occasionally results are significant at the 0.001 (0.1%) significance level, which is very significant indeed. Even when this happens it does not *prove* that there is a real effect. It means that we should provisionally accept the idea of a real difference rather than suppose that a very improbable chance result has occurred.

16. Simple tests with *z*

INTRODUCTION

The ideas of significance tests can be extended to various practical situations. This chapter, and the 5 which follow it, will show you how to apply significance tests to:

1. Large samples where the data are quantitative (in this chapter).
2. Small samples where the data are quantitative (in the next chapter).
3. The correlation coefficients (in Chapter 18).
4. Results from a regression analysis (in Chapter 19).
5. Qualitative data (in Chapter 20).
6. Data which are not assumed to follow any particular distribution (in Chapter 21).

Further ideas used in this chapter involve the distribution of $\bar{x}$ and $(\bar{x}_1 - \bar{x}_2)$, and z. Re-read the summaries of Chapters 12 and 14 if your memory is rusty and if necessary re-read the two chapters completely.

16.1	What are the stages in significance testing?	State the Null Hypothesis and its alternative. Calculate *p*. Draw conclusions.
16.2	We are going to test the following results. Ms Bright wants to know whether the I.Q. of children with bilharzia is lower than normal. She uses an intelligence test which has been so designed as to give a population mean of 100 with a standard deviation 12. She finds that her random sample of 36 students with bilharzia have a mean result of 96. State the Null Hypothesis and its alternative.	The Null Hypothesis is that any experimental difference is only due to chance variation, and the alternative is that children with bilharzia have a lower I.Q. than normal.
	This test involves .... tail(s).	one We are not testing whether they have a higher I.Q.
16.3	We initially assume that the .... is true.	Null Hypothesis

16.4 This being so, we can initially assume that children with bilharzia are no different from the general population, so far as their I.Q. is concerned. Therefore, Ms Bright's value $\bar{x}$ can be assumed to have been taken at random from the general distribution of $\bar{x}$. Complete the general distribution of $\bar{x}$, the sample mean.

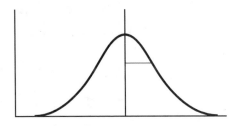

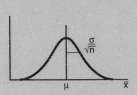

16.5 What is the other name and what is the symbol for its standard deviation?

The standard error of the mean, $s_{\bar{x}}$ (the sample estimate of the population value)

16.6 Sketch the specific distribution of $\bar{x}$ drawn from the population in Frame 16.2 using the values for μ, σ and n given there.

$\mu = 100$, $\sigma = 12$, $n = 36$

$$\therefore \frac{\sigma}{\sqrt{n}} = \frac{12}{\sqrt{36}} = 2$$

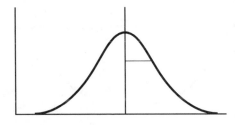

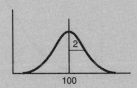

16.7 Mark in Ms Bright's result $\bar{x}$.
How many standard errors away from the mean is it?
What is its z value?

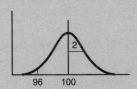

It is 2 standard errors below the mean so the z value is -2.

16.8   We can check that $z = -2$.
Complete this formula for calculating z:

$$z = \frac{\text{the result} - (a)}{(b)}$$

(a) The mean
(b) The standard deviation

16.9   For the distribution of $\bar{x}$ in general:

The mean = ?

The standard deviation = ?

The mean = μ

The standard deviation

$$= \frac{\sigma}{\sqrt{n}}$$

z = ?

$$z = \frac{\bar{x} - \mu}{\dfrac{\sigma}{\sqrt{n}}}$$

16.10   Substituting the results from Frame 16.2
directly in this equation we calculate z = ?
This is a simple example of what is
called a test statistic.

$$\frac{96 - 100}{\dfrac{12}{\sqrt{36}}} = \frac{-4}{2}$$

$$= -2 \text{ again}$$

16.11   Mark Ms Bright's result on the *standard
normal curve*.

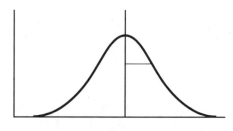

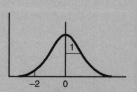

16.12   What is the next step in performing any
significance test?

Calculate p.

16.13   What does p represent?

The probability of the
result or a more extreme
result arising by chance

16.14   Look at Frame 16.2 again. Is Ms Bright
interested in both ends of the scale?

No – only the end where
her sample I.Q. is *lower*
than normal

16.15 Shade the equivalent p area in this test (using the results in Frame 16.11).

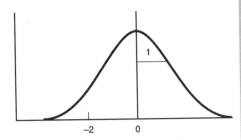

16.16 What is the size of the area equivalent to this value p?
The diagram in Frame 14.5 is repeated here.

0.025 (2$\frac{1}{2}$%)
(approximately)
(More precisely it is 0.023 (2.3%).)

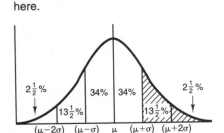

16.17 Confirm this result from the tables relating p to z on page 274. The p value there refers to one/two end(s) of the distribution.

two
p = 0.05, approximately, (past z = 2) at both ends together.
p = 0.025, approximately, (past z = −2) at one end.

16.18 p = 0.025, approximately, in this significance test. Is 0.05 > p > 0.01?

Yes

16.19 What conclusion does Ms Bright draw?

The result is significantly lower at the 0.05 (5%) significance level.
On the basis of those particular results it appears that children with bilharzia have a significantly lower I.Q. at this level of significance.

16.19   *cont'd*

(N.B. Significance tests say nothing about whether bilharzia *causes* the lower I.Q., only that there is in fact a relationship. Those with lower I.Q.'s may actually have been more likely to contract the disease by swimming in infected water.) There is as yet insufficient evidence for a significant difference at the 0.01 (1%) significance level.
Note. Had a two-tailed test been appropriate here, the result would have been right on the boundary of significance at the 0.05 (5%) level. Strictly speaking the result would have been just significant at the 5% level (since the precise *p* value is 0.046). But this is a good example of a case where it is more informative to quote a *p* value, rather than just the outcome of a significance test. This also illustrates how an unscrupulous worker could 'turn' a marginal, or even a non-significant result, on a two-tailed test into a significant result on a one-tailed test. Watch out for this whenever you see one-tailed tests being used.

16.20   You have completed your first significance test using '*z*'. As the magnitude of *z* gets bigger the *p* value gets ....

smaller (The exception to this arises when testing, for example, a Null Hypothesis such as $\mu = 0$ against an Alternative Hypothesis that $\mu < 0$, and when the observed sample mean $\bar{x}$ turns out to be > 0, i.e. in the opposite direction to what is expected when stating the Alternative Hypothesis.)

16.20 *cont'd*

Note the importance of the phrase 'the magnitude of' here. In this particular example, large-in-magnitude negative values of z are associated with small p values.

16.21 The Null Hypothesis is rejected if p is bigger/smaller than the significance level. Therefore the Null Hypothesis is rejected if the magnitude of z you calculated from the results is bigger/smaller than the significant value of z.
That is:

smaller

bigger

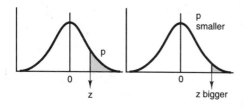

Note that the example illustrated in the diagram corresponds to the case where the interest is in the upper tail of the distribution only (so constituting a one-tailed test), rather than the lower tail as in the preceding frames concerning the bilharzia/I.Q. examples.

16.22 If Ms Bright had not known μ she would have estimated it using the mean of a .... sample.

control

16.23 Of what would her control sample have consisted?

A random sample of similar children without bilharzia

16.24 If Ms Bright had not known σ she could have calculated .... instead.

s
This is the sample standard deviation, which can be used as an estimate of the population standard deviation.

16.25 State a formula she might have used.

$$s = \sqrt{\frac{\Sigma(x - \bar{x})^2}{n - 1}}$$

$$\text{or } \sqrt{\frac{\Sigma(x^2) - \frac{(\Sigma x)^2}{n}}{n - 1}}$$

16.26 Look at the following survey results. State the Null Hypothesis and its alternative.
Ms Bright wants to know whether there is any difference in the mean weight of children aged 8 years with bilharzia compared with those without.
She calculated the mean weight of a random sample of 50 bilharzial children as 27.4 kg and of a random sample of 50 non-bilharzial children as 28.2 kg. The standard deviation for all the children is known to be 2.3 kg.

The Null Hypothesis states that any difference is due to chance whereas its alternative is that children with bilharzia have a different weight from normal children.

16.27 Assuming the Null Hypothesis is true, the sample of children with bilharzia and her control are presumed to come from populations with the same ....

means

16.28 The difference between the bilharzial sample mean and the control sample mean follows which distribution?

The distribution of the difference between two sample means

16.29 Complete the following distribution (the distribution of the difference between two sample means) in general terms, assuming a common variance for the populations from which the samples are taken.

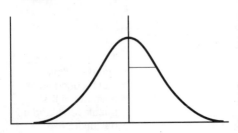

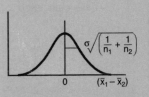

16.29 *cont'd*

Note that in general the two samples may be taken from populations with unequal variances, σ_1^2 and σ_2^2, say. The variance of the difference between the two sample means is then

$\dfrac{\sigma_1^2}{n_1} + \dfrac{\sigma_2^2}{n_2}$, and the standard

deviation (i.e. the standard error of the difference) is

$$\sqrt{\dfrac{\sigma_1^2}{n_1} + \dfrac{\sigma_2^2}{n_2}}.$$

Of course, this reduces to

$$\sigma\sqrt{\dfrac{1}{n_1} + \dfrac{1}{n_2}} \quad \text{when}$$

$\sigma_1 = \sigma_2 = \sigma.$

16.30 What is the value of

$$\sigma\sqrt{\dfrac{1}{n_1} + \dfrac{1}{n_2}}$$

using the data in Frame 16.26?

$2.3\sqrt{\dfrac{1}{50} + \dfrac{1}{50}} = 2.3\sqrt{\dfrac{1}{25}} = 0.46$

16.31 What is the value of $(\bar{x}_1 - \bar{x}_2)$ in Frame 16.26? (Call children with bilharzia the 1st sample and the control group the 2nd.)

-0.8 kg

16.32 This value is just one of many possible values of $(\bar{x}_1 - \bar{x}_2)$ under the Null Hypothesis. How many standard deviations is it from the mean?

$-0.8/0.46 = -1.74$
That is its z value.

16.33 What is the formula for calculating z using the distribution of the difference between two sample means? (Refer back to Frame 14.55 if you need to.)

$$z = \dfrac{\bar{x}_1 - \bar{x}_2}{\sigma\sqrt{\left[\dfrac{1}{n_1} + \dfrac{1}{n_2}\right]}}$$

If σ is unknown, but we have an estimate s of it, we have:

$$z = \dfrac{\bar{x}_1 - \bar{x}_2}{s\sqrt{\left[\dfrac{1}{n_1} + \dfrac{1}{n_2}\right]}},$$

16.33 *cont'd*

though, strictly speaking, the statistic is no longer z, but t (see below).

We will see in a later frame how we combine estimates s_1^2 and s_2^2 of the unknown variance σ^2 from two separate samples, leading to an overall estimate s^2 of σ^2.

But then we need to use a t test, rather than a z test (see the next chapter). However, if the samples are both large, i.e. of size 30 or more, a z test instead provides a satisfactory approximation.

16.34 What is z calculated to be from the data in Frame 16.26?

$$z = \frac{-0.8}{2.3\sqrt{\frac{1}{50} + \frac{1}{50}}} = -1.74$$

i.e. the same result as before.

16.35 Ms Bright in Frame 16.26 is concerned with one/two tails, so the significance level applies to one/two tails?

two

two (You can use the table in this book directly, but remember, if you are using other tables, you must check what is being tabulated.)

16.36 What is the equivalent significant value of z using the tables relating z to p on page 274.
(a) if the significance level is 0.05 (5%)?

(a) For 0.05, the significant value of $z = 1.96$ (= 2.0, rounding to one decimal place). (This is often referred to as the *critical value*.)

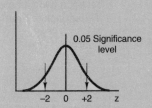

0.05 Significance level

−2   0   +2   z

16.36 *cont'd*
(b) if the significance level is 0.01 (1%)?

(b) For 0.01, the significant value (critical value) of $z = 2.57$ ($= 2.6$, rounding to one decimal place).
That is:

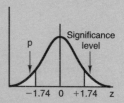

16.37 We decided that we would reject the Null Hypothesis if the z calculated from the results is bigger in magnitude than the significant value (critical value) of z.
Here, calculated $z = -1.74$, and
significant $z = 1.96$ (0.05) or 2.57 (0.01).

Sketch this idea.

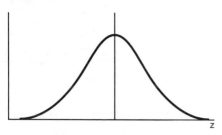

What is your conclusion?

We accept the Null Hypothesis. Either there is no difference or there is insufficient evidence to indicate a difference.

Note that it is always sensible to draw a diagram of what is going on. This is especially so if you are at all confused about what you are doing – the diagram should help to clarify your thinking.

16.38 Your calculated value of z from the experiment was bigger/smaller in magnitude than the equivalent significant value (critical value) z, so p was bigger/smaller than the significance level and so the Null Hypothesis was not rejected.

smaller

bigger

16.39 If you know the value of μ you do/do not need a control sample, and under the Null Hypothesis the sample mean follows which distribution?

do not
The distribution of sample means – a normal distribution

16.40   Under what condition?

If the sample is random and fairly large

16.41   Then z can be calculated using which formula?

$$z = \frac{\bar{x} - \mu}{\dfrac{\sigma}{\sqrt{n}}}$$

16.42   If you do not know μ you can estimate it from a control sample and then

$z = ?$

$$\frac{\bar{x}_1 - \bar{x}_2}{\sigma\sqrt{\left[\dfrac{1}{n_1} + \dfrac{1}{n_2}\right]}}$$

or $\dfrac{\bar{x}_1 - \bar{x}_2}{s\sqrt{\left[\dfrac{1}{n_1} + \dfrac{1}{n_2}\right]}}$

when σ is not known.

You should recognise these from the formulae that were presented in Frame 16.33 for the case of the difference between two sample means.

16.43   When you do not know σ use ....

s from the samples (but see Frames 16.44 and 17.50 to put this into context).

16.44   There are different values of s^2 (s_1^2 and s_2^2, say) from the two samples, which may in general be taken from populations with different variances σ_1^2 and σ_2^2, respectively (see the note on Frame 16.29). s_1^2 is an estimate of σ_1^2, and s_2^2 is an estimate of σ_2^2, so what is the estimate of the standard error of the difference between the sample means,

$$\sqrt{\frac{\sigma_1^2}{n_1} + \frac{\sigma_2^2}{n_2}} \; ?$$

The estimate is $\sqrt{\dfrac{s_1^2}{n_1} + \dfrac{s_2^2}{n_2}}$.

16.45   Look at this survey.
Professor Trunk wishes to know whether there is any difference in width of a particular thoracic vertebra between different ethnic groups. He measures,

16.45 *cont'd*
using a standardised X-ray procedure, the relevant width on the random samples of 64 Zambians and 32 Mozambicans. For the Zambians the mean width was 7.31 units (variance 0.06) and for the Mozambicans the mean was 7.16 units (variance 0.05). Perform the necessary test by completing the schedule below.
State the Null Hypothesis.

The difference is only due to chance.

State its alternative.

There is a significant difference between the widths.

16.46 Under the Null Hypothesis these particular experimental results follow which distribution?

The difference between two sample means – a normal distribution

16.47 You do not know σ_1^2 and σ_2^2 so you calculate s_1^2 and s_2^2 and use z = (formula)?

$$z = \frac{\bar{x}_1 - \bar{x}_2}{\sqrt{\dfrac{s_1^2}{n_1} + \dfrac{s_2^2}{n_2}}}$$

equivalent to (an estimate of):

$$z = \frac{\bar{x}_1 - \bar{x}_2}{\sqrt{\dfrac{\sigma_1^2}{n_1} + \dfrac{\sigma_2^2}{n_2}}}$$

16.48 Therefore z here = ... (value)

$$\frac{7.31 - 7.16}{\sqrt{\dfrac{0.06}{64} + \dfrac{0.05}{32}}} = \frac{0.15}{\sqrt{\dfrac{0.16}{64}}} = 3$$

16.49 Professor Trunk is interested in .... tail(s).
The equivalent z value to the commonly used significance levels are (see the table) =

two
1.96 for a significance level of 0.05, 2.57 for a significance level of 0.01

16.50 The calculated z from the experiment is bigger/smaller in magnitude than the significant value (critical value) of z, and

bigger

16.50 *cont'd*

p is therefore bigger/smaller than the significance level.

Hence the conclusion is

....

....

....

smaller
(At the 0.01 (1%) significance level.)

That there is a significant difference between Zambians and Mozambicans with respect to thoracic vertebra width ($p < 0.01$), the Zambians having, on average, the larger vertebra width.
Note that the two sample variances in this example did not differ from each other by very much, and it would have been reasonable to have assumed a common underlying population variance, and to have used a pooled estimate s^2 of it. We will see in the next chapter that this is the approach that we adopt in small samples, leading to a t test. However, in this example we have been able to use a test based on z (so based on the normal distribution) as a good approximation to the true statistic, because the samples were large (both containing more than 30 observations) and we have not needed to make the common variance assumption.

16.51 **Practical example**

Repeat the format in the previous frame to decide whether the means here are significantly different.

Dr Adder wanted to know whether inclusion of B_{12} in guinea pig diets increased the weight gain. After a fixed period he found the mean weight gain of

See page 256.

16.51   *cont'd*
         50 randomly chosen guinea pigs without
         B_{12} was 148 g ($s = 40$ g) and of 50
         randomly chosen guinea pigs given B_{12}
         was 156 g ($s = 37$ g).

16.52   You are possibly concerned about the
         tie-up between the *significance levels*,
         0.05 and 0.01, and *p* on the one hand,
         and the *significant value* (*critical
         value*) of *z* and *calculated z* on the
         other.
         Does this diagram help?

Yes – we hope so.
The significance levels
0.05 and 0.01 correspond
to the significant value
(critical value) of *z*. *p* and
calculated *z* relate to the
actual results calculated
from the data.

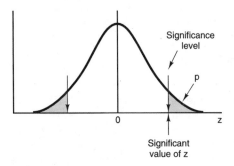

16.53   The experimental results themselves
         provide a value *z* called 'calculated *z*'. It
         is a measure of how extreme your
         particular result is, if the Null Hypothesis
         is ....

true

16.54   *p* is the probability of such an
         extreme, or a more extreme, value of
         calculated *z* occurring by chance.
         The value of *p* increases as the
         corresponding calculated *z*
         ....

decreases (in
magnitude)
(But see the note in
Frame 16.20 on the
exception, bearing in
mind that the directions
are now the other way
round.)

16.55 That is,

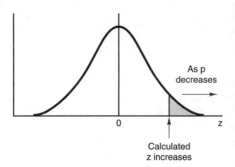

As p
decreases
→

0   z

Calculated
z increases

You reject the Null Hypothesis if p is
smaller/greater than the significance
level, i.e. if the calculated z is
smaller/greater in magnitude than the
significant value (critical value) of z.

smaller

greater

16.56 Four conditions for applying z tests
should be satisfied before they can be
used. They are:

a) The sample must be chosen ....

randomly

b) The data must be
qualitative/quantitative.

quantitative

c) The variable must be distributed in
the population ....

normally (although this
approximation is not so
important, in fact, if the
samples are particularly
large).

d) The sizes of the samples must be 30
or greater. (There is one exception
we will mention again in the next
chapter.)

16.57 We have used z tests on the data in
Frames:

16.2
16.26
16.45
16.51

Were all these conditions satisfied?

Yes

16.58 In the next chapter we will solve
problems where small samples are
involved but the three conditions
otherwise are as for z tests.
State them.

Random samples
Quantitative data
Normal distribution of the
variable being considered

SUMMARY

Simple tests involving 'z' are used:
1. When the samples are random.
2. When the data are quantitative.
3. When the variable can be assumed to be normally distributed in the population.
4. Usually when the samples involved are bigger in size than 30.

A. *To test the difference between a sample mean and a known value of* μ:

Here $z = \dfrac{\bar{x} - \mu}{\dfrac{s}{\sqrt{n}}}$ or $\dfrac{\bar{x} - \mu}{\dfrac{\sigma}{\sqrt{n}}}$ if σ is known.

B. *To test the difference between two sample means or a sample mean and a control mean:*

Here $z = \dfrac{(\bar{x}_1 - \bar{x}_2)}{\sqrt{\dfrac{s_1^2}{n_1} + \dfrac{s_2^2}{n_2}}}$

or $\dfrac{(\bar{x}_1 - \bar{x}_2)}{\sqrt{\dfrac{\sigma_1^2}{n_1} + \dfrac{\sigma_2^2}{n_2}}}$ if σ_1^2 and σ_2^2 are known.

If the populations from which the samples are taken have a common variance then this last expression becomes $\dfrac{(\bar{x}_1 - \bar{x}_2)}{\sigma\sqrt{\dfrac{1}{n_1} + \dfrac{1}{n_2}}}$.

As the calculated value of z increases in magnitude, p, the probability of a more extreme value by chance, decreases. (The exception to this arises in a one-tailed test, when the observed result is in the opposite direction to the alternative hypothesis.)

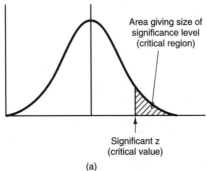

Area giving size of significance level (critical region)

Significant z (critical value)

(a)

Summary *cont'd*

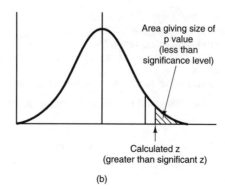

(b)

The Null Hypothesis is rejected if *p* is *smaller* than the significance level. This is equivalent to the value of *z* calculated from the results being *greater* in magnitude than the particular significant value (critical value) of *z*.

Note. One of the conditions for using *z* tests has been presented here as being when the samples involved are bigger in size than 30. (In fact, if σ is known – which is not usually the case – the approach is valid, even for small samples, provided that the variable itself has a normal distribution.) But the approach is then really an approximation to the correct approach, involving the *t* distribution, which we will meet in the next chapter. So in the above, wherever a formula for *z* involves *s*, or s_1 and s_2, the result is only approximate, and the *t* distribution provides the more strictly correct approach. Now, the normal distribution is more extensively tabulated than the *t* distribution, so when tests tended to be carried out by hand, there was a desire to use normal distribution tables whenever possible. Historically, then, a distinction was made between large and small samples for the use of *z* and *t* tests, respectively. But in an age now where exact *p* values from such standard distributions can be generated easily by a computer, such a distinction is largely redundant, and is therefore rarely made. Particular importance therefore attaches to the next chapter.

17. Simple tests with Student's *t*

INTRODUCTION

The method for significance testing when the samples are smaller than 30, say (but see the note at the end of the last chapter), was discovered by a man called William Sealy Gosset in 1908. At the time he was employed by the Guinness brewery in Dublin. The firm's regulations required him to use a pen-name and he chose the name 'Student'; '*t*' was the symbol later introduced in connection with the distribution used, which is consequently known as 'Student's *t* distribution'.

17.1 What are the criteria for using *z* in a one-sample test?

Random samples. Quantitative data. Normal distribution. Sample size at least 30.

17.2 Occasionally you can use the *z* tests even if *n* is less than 30. The requirement is that σ is known accurately and not estimated using ....

s

17.3 If *n* is less than 30 and σ is unknown, *t* tests are required.
Complete this table of tests to be used:

	n < 30	*n* = 30 or more
σ known	?	*z*
σ unknown	?	?

z *z*
t *z*
(In fact, *t* can be used whenever σ is unknown; but when *n* is bigger than 30, the *t* distribution becomes so like the *z* distribution (i.e. the standard normal distribution) that *z* can be used instead. But there is nothing really to be gained from this – it is better really to use *t* whenever σ is unknown. See the note at the end of the last chapter.)

17.4	The criteria for using t are otherwise the same as for z. State the criteria for using t tests.	Random samples. Quantitative data. Normal distribution. Sample size less than 30 and σ unknown. (This last criterion can be simplified to just 'σ unknown', so that we forget about the possibility of using the normal distribution as an approximation to the t distribution – just use the exact procedure instead.)
17.5	When t is used we never use .... but s^2.	σ^2
17.6	State the formula for calculating s^2.	$s^2 = \sqrt{\dfrac{\Sigma(x - \bar{x})^2}{n - 1}}$, or $s^2 = \dfrac{\Sigma(x^2) - \dfrac{(\Sigma x)^2}{n}}{n - 1}$
17.7	Here is an example. Would you use t or z? Why? Dr Chest is interested in knowing whether people who have had heart attacks have a blood cholesterol level different from the normal level of 180 mg/100 ml. He has a random sample of 16 patients and calculates their mean blood cholesterol as 195 mg/100 ml with a variance of 900 mg²/100 ml.	t Random sample. Quantitative data. Blood cholesterol levels can be assumed to follow the normal distribution in the population. n is less than 30 and σ is unknown.
17.8	What are the stages in performing a significance test?	a) State the Null Hypothesis and its alternative. b) Calculate p (using z or t, as appropriate). c) Draw conclusions.
17.9	Perform the first stage for the data in Frame 17.7.	The Null Hypothesis is that the difference is only due to chance.

17.9   *cont'd*

The alternative is that people surviving heart attacks have a different blood cholesterol level.

17.10   A *t* distribution is very like the standard normal distribution. The formula for calculating *t* is very similar to that for calculating ....

z

17.11 μ in Frame 17.7 is known. Therefore if 30 or more patients had been used which formula would you have used for *z*?

(Look back to the summary at the end of Chapter 16 if your memory is failing you.)

$z = \dfrac{\bar{x} - \mu}{\dfrac{\sigma}{\sqrt{n}}}$ if σ is known.

But, as σ is not known in this example,

$z = \dfrac{\bar{x} - \mu}{\dfrac{s}{\sqrt{n}}}$

Now, as we have seen earlier, when σ is unknown and *s* is used instead, this formula is just an approximation to the exact result, which is $t = \dfrac{\bar{x} - \mu}{\dfrac{s}{\sqrt{n}}}$.

17.12   Following on from 17.11, $t = \dfrac{\bar{x} - \mu}{\dfrac{s}{\sqrt{n}}}$.

It does not equal $\dfrac{\bar{x} - \mu}{\dfrac{\sigma}{\sqrt{n}}}$. Why not?

Because, if σ is known, *t* would not be used. (The formula would then be for *z*, not *t*.)

17.13   What is the value of *t* in Frame 17.7?

$s^2 = 900$, $\therefore s = 30$ and

$t = \dfrac{195 - 180}{\dfrac{30}{\sqrt{16}}} = \dfrac{15}{7\frac{1}{2}} = +2$

17.14	The calculated value of t is 2. The next problem is to find the .... of t.	significant value (critical value)
17.15	This is not so straightforward as for z, because there are a series of t distributions which cannot all be standardised to one t distribution. They all depend on the symbol f, the number of degrees of freedom. f equals the value of the denominator when s^2 is calculated. What value has f in Frame 17.7?	$f = 15$ because $$s^2 = \frac{\sum(x - \bar{x})^2}{n - 1}$$ $$= \frac{\sum(x - \bar{x})^2}{15}$$ here. So 15 is the value of the denominator.
17.16	The significant value (critical value) of t which you require is that where .... = 15.	f
17.17	The t tables, like the z table, include the area in one/two tails?	Two. (In this book, at least. Again, when using other tables you must be careful to check exactly what is being tabulated.)
17.18	In Frame 17.7 Dr Chest is interested in one/two tails?	two
17.19	Therefore you need the significant value (critical value) of t when $f = 15$ in the columns of the significance levels for 2 tails. Look at the t tables on page 279. What is the required significant value (critical value) of t?	2.131 for 0.05 (5%) significance level 2.947 for 0.01 (1%) significance level
17.20	The conclusions for calculated and significant t follow in the same way as they would have done had we calculated z and looked up a significant value (critical value) of z. What is your conclusion here?	In both cases the calculated t is less than the significant t (critical value). You accept the Null Hypothesis. Your conclusion is either that there is no real difference, or that there is a real difference, but insufficient evidence to show it.

17.20 *cont'd*

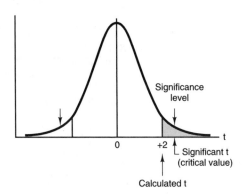

17.21 Do you remember how you could distinguish between these two conclusions?

Yes, we hope so. You would make *n* bigger.

17.22 Dr Clever Dick tells Dr Chest that in fact he should only have tested to see whether the blood cholesterol level was higher than normal. (The literature excludes the possibility of its being lower.) The test then would include one/two tails?

one only

17.23 Remember that the main headings of the *t* tables on page 279 include both tails. What are the significant values (critical values) of *t* now?

1.753 for 0.05 (5%) significance level
2.602 for 0.01 (1%) significance level

17.24 Dr Clever Dick's conclusion, if he had been performing this experiment, would have been what?
(Remember we calculated *t* to be 2.)

He would have accepted the alternative as true at the 0.05 (5%) level but not at the 0.01 (1%) level ($0.01 < p < 0.05$).
This indicates how significance tests are made more sensitive if one-tailed tests can be used. But, again, note also how this approach can be abused by the unscrupulous investigator – and beware! Look out for the trick of using a one-

| 17.24 | *cont'd* | tailed test (when it is not appropriate) just to obtain a significant result. So, although someone may be 'clever' to obtain a significant result, he may also be dishonest in doing so, by using an inappropriate test procedure. |

17.25 When $n = 20$, $f =$ ....

19

17.26 As f gets bigger, the t distribution becomes more nearly normal, until when $f =$ ...., we can safely use z tables instead of t.

$f = 29$
($n = 30$)
When f is infinitely large the t distribution is exactly the same as the standard normal distribution. Of course, you can see from inspection of tabulated values from the distributions, just how different the two distributions are for finite values of n.

17.27 f represents what is called the number of degrees of freedom (or free choices). A playing captain wants to choose the rest of his hockey team.
In statistical symbols
.... = 11
(symbol)

$n = 11$

.... = 10

$f = 10$
Because the captain is playing, he only has 10 'degrees of freedom' (free choices).

17.28 This should give you some idea why statisticians call 'f' the 'number of degrees of freedom'.

z does not use $s^2 / \sigma^2 / f$.

z never uses f.
Also, strictly speaking, z does not use s^2 (though t

17.28 *cont'd*

does). But for large samples, z can provide a good approximation to t, even when using s^2 (though you may choose to use t still, as is strictly correct).

t does not use $s^2 / \sigma^2 / f$.

t never uses σ^2.

17.29 What are the criteria for using t tests?

Random samples.
Quantitative data.
Normal distribution.
n less than 30 and σ not known.
(Or, this last criterion can be simplified to 'σ not known'.)

17.30 Although t tests can be used to analyse results from very small samples these tests on mini-samples are not very sensitive.
However, for the sake of practice, imagine here that the results refer to the pain threshold for only 5 randomly selected patients after administration of a new analgesic. Are these results significantly higher than the population average, 4 units?
Also, for practice, assume the pain thresholds are approximately normally distributed. (You can see that this is an approximation because the pain thresholds are apparently discrete data.)

Patient	A	B	C	D	E
Pain threshold	7	5	2	4	7

$\bar{x} =$

$s^2 =$

$\therefore s =$

$\bar{x} = 5$

$$s^2 = \frac{\Sigma(x - \bar{x})^2}{n - 1}$$

$$= \frac{4 + 0 + 9 + 1 + 4}{4} = 4\frac{1}{2}$$

$s \simeq 2.1$

172

17.30 *cont'd*
and $f =$

$f = 4$ (the denominator when s^2 is calculated)

$n =$

$n = 5$

$\mu =$

$\mu = 4$

Calculated $t = \dfrac{\bar{x} - \mu}{\dfrac{s}{\sqrt{n}}}$

$t = \dfrac{5 - 4}{\dfrac{2.1}{\sqrt{5}}} \simeq 1$

$= ?$

This is a .... tailed test with f equal to .... so the corresponding significant values (critical values) of $t =$ What is your conclusion?

one-
4
2.132 for the 0.05 (5%) level
3.747 for the 0.01 (1%) level

The calculated t is less than the significant (critical) t at both the above levels. So we still accept the Null Hypothesis. The analgesic is either ineffective or there is insufficient evidence to show otherwise. (Of course, with only 5 patients it is highly likely that the sample is too small to show the difference anyway, even if one truly exists.)

17.31 Look at these results.
A psychiatrist got exasperated when patients phoned him during the night (waking him up!) to complain of insomnia. He heard of a new drug 'Zizz' and decided to try it randomly on 5 patients to see whether it was effective. He gave them alternately at random a placebo for a week and Zizz for a week and calculated the average number of hours per night each patient slept while receiving the placebo and while receiving Zizz.

17.31 *cont'd*
Here are the results:

	Average time on placebo (hrs)	Average time on Zizz (hrs)
Patient A	2	7
Patient B	6	13
Patient C	3	6
Patient D	1	0
Patient E	4	5

Incidentally, Patient B lost his job!

The results can be modified so that *t* can be used. The pairs of results are subtracted so that *x* (in the terminology of the previous frame) now refers to these differences. This modification is consequently called the paired *t*-test (on differences).

Fill in the missing values.

Patient	Average time on placebo (hrs)	Average time on Zizz (hrs)	Difference (hrs)
A	2	7	+5
B	6	13	+7
C	3	6	(a)
D	1	0	(b)
E	4	5	+1

(a) = +3
(b) = −1

17.32 These *differences* between the two drugs are based on a .... sample of patients, the data are ...., and we assume that the differences are approximately .... distributed. *n* equals ...., and σ is/is not known.

random
quantitative

normally
5 (the number of differences)
Is not

17.33 Therefore we can use a .... test on these *differences.* We treat these differences 5, 7, 3, −1, 1, as 5 values of a variable.

t

17.34 Perform the first stage.

The Null Hypothesis is that the differences are only due to chance. The alternative is that Zizz increases the average number of hours sleep.

17.35 We are going to perform the *t* test using these 5 differences (called *x* below). Complete the table and calculate $\bar{x}$ and *s* for these differences.

Patient	x	$(x - \bar{x})$	$(x - \bar{x})^2$
A	5	2	4
B	7	4	16
C	3		
D	-1	-4	
E	+1		

$\sum x = $ $\sum (x - \bar{x}) = 0$ $\sum (x - \bar{x})^2 = $
of course

Patient	x	$(x - \bar{x})$	$(x - \bar{x})^2$
A	5	2	4
B	7	4	16
C	3	0	0
D	-1	-4	16
E	+1	-2	4

$\sum x = 15$ $\sum (x - \bar{x})^2 = 40$

$$\bar{x} = \frac{\sum x}{n} = ?$$

$$s = \sqrt{\frac{\sum (x - \bar{x})^2}{n - 1}} = ?$$

$$\bar{x} = \frac{15}{5} = 3$$

$$s = \sqrt{\frac{\sum (x - \bar{x})^2}{n - 1}}$$

$$= \sqrt{\frac{40}{4}}$$

$$= \sqrt{10}$$

17.36 $\therefore f = ?$

$f = n - 1 = 4$

17.37 Under the Null Hypothesis there is no real difference and so theoretically the mean difference should equal ....

0, i.e. $\mu = 0$

17.38 We use the same formula here as before.

$\therefore t =$

$$t = \frac{\bar{x} - \mu}{\dfrac{s}{\sqrt{n}}}$$

(Frame 17.12, if you had forgotten.)

17.39   In this example

$\bar{x}$ = ? (Frame 17.35)
μ = ? (Frame 17.37)
s = ? (Frame 17.35)
n = ? (the number of differences)

∴ Calculated t =

$\bar{x} = 3$
$\mu = 0$
$s = \sqrt{10}$
$n = 5$

$$\frac{3 - 0}{\dfrac{\sqrt{10}}{\sqrt{5}}} = \frac{3}{\sqrt{2}} \simeq 2.12$$

17.40   Calculated $t = 2.12$.
The psychiatrist is interested in one/two tail(s).
The significant (critical) value of t = ($f = 4$, remember).

One. He wants to know whether the drug is more effective than the placebo.
2.132 for the 0.05 (5%) level
3.747 for the 0.01 (1%) level

17.41   The calculated t is .... than the significant (critical) value of t. Therefore we accept/reject the Null Hypothesis.

smaller in magnitude

accept

Note, however, that the calculated value of t is only just less than the significant (critical) value of t at the 5% level. The result is therefore almost significant at that level. This illustrates clearly the merit of quoting a p value for a test, rather than just stating whether the result is significant or not, and hence whether the null hypothesis is rejected or not.

17.42   Such tests based on the differences between pairs of results on individuals are called paired t-tests. In paired t-tests suppose that the variable is x and that we therefore use

$$t = \frac{\bar{x} - \mu}{\dfrac{s}{\sqrt{n}}}$$

What do these symbols mean in the context of paired t-tests?

x is the difference between each of the paired results.
$\bar{x}$ is the mean of the *differences*.
μ is the theoretical mean *difference* = 0.
s is the standard deviation for these *differences*.
n is the number of *differences*.

17.43 Pairing results is a good idea if the results fall naturally into pairs, i.e. each member is more closely related to its pair than any other result. The natural variability in the data is then mainly the variability that you are interested in (e.g. in a comparison between treatments) rather than being mixed up with variability that you are not so interested in (e.g. between subjects).

You have a series of twins. You should/should not arrange to treat the results in pairs.

should
A twin is more like its twin than any other person.

17.44 Noah, in his ark, had he had the time (or the inclination!) to do a drug trial on his animals, should/should not have used the paired *t*-test?

should

17.45 When would you pair?

When the two members of each of the pairs are more like one another than the rest of the group.

17.46 Most frequently the paired *t*-test is used when two drugs are given to each patient or when a specimen is tested using two different techniques. When results fall naturally into pairs we can treat the .... as the variable and straightaway use

differences

$$t = \frac{\bar{x} - \mu}{\dfrac{s}{\sqrt{n}}}$$

where $\mu = ?$

0

17.47 Give two experimental situations where you would use the paired *t*-test
a)
b)

For example:
a) Twins
b) A drug trial with 'before' and 'after' results
c) In animal experiments where two animals are taken from each litter
d) Some doctors match patients successfully for age/sex/severity of

17.47 *cont'd*

disease but if the matched people are not very alike this can be a mistake
e) In comparing two chemical analytical methods
f) A trial comparing two different skin treatments, which can be applied to different limbs of the same person

17.48 To recap from the last chapter:
When z is used and μ is unknown we standardise the distribution of ....
....
....
....
and use the formula:
$z = $ ...., in the case where we can assume equal variances for the underlying populations.

the difference between two sample means (one of which is from the control group usually)

$$z = \frac{\bar{x}_1 - \bar{x}_2}{\sigma \sqrt{\dfrac{1}{n_1} + \dfrac{1}{n_2}}}.$$

17.49 When t is used and μ is unknown – and now the common standard deviation σ is unknown as well – instead of using

$$z = \frac{\bar{x}_1 - \bar{x}_2}{\sigma \sqrt{\dfrac{1}{n_1} + \dfrac{1}{n_2}}}$$

you can imagine we use $t = ?$

σ is replaced by s, to give:

$$t = \frac{\bar{x}_1 - \bar{x}_2}{s \sqrt{\dfrac{1}{n_1} + \dfrac{1}{n_2}}}.$$

Remember, a combined estimate s^2 of σ^2 can be derived from the separate sample variances, s_1^2 and s_2^2 (equal variances in the populations assumed).

17.50 We have to modify our usual formula for s^2 so as to include the results from both samples. As we saw in Chapter 16, when using the standard normal distribution we could use each of the s_1^2, s_2^2 values separately as in the following form of the z statistic:

17.50   *cont'd*

$$z = \frac{\bar{x}_1 - \bar{x}_2}{\sqrt{\dfrac{s_1^2}{n_1} + \dfrac{s_2^2}{n_2}}}.$$

As has already been indicated, when we use the *t* distribution we assume equal variances in the populations from which the two samples are taken, and construct an estimate, s^2, of the unknown variance, σ^2, by pooling the squares of the deviations from the means, as follows:

1st sample   2nd sample

$$s^2 = \frac{\Sigma(x_1 - \bar{x}_1)^2 + \Sigma(x_2 - \bar{x}_2)^2}{n_1 - 1 \quad + \quad n_2 - 1}$$

Which formula for s^2, which you are used to, is this pooled formula most like?

$$s^2 = \frac{\Sigma(x - \bar{x})^2}{n - 1}$$

17.51   Using the result of the previous frame, express the pooled estimate of variance, s^2, in terms of s_1^2, s_2^2, n_1 and n_2.

$$s^2 = \frac{(n_1 - 1)s_1^2 + (n_2 - 1)s_2^2}{n_1 - 1 + n_2 - 1}$$

$$= \frac{(n_1 - 1)s_1^2 + (n_2 - 1)s_2^2}{n_1 + n_2 - 2}$$

17.52   Let us take an over-simplified example.

Suppose the 1st sample is 1, 2, 3:

x_1	$(x_1 - \bar{x}_1)$	$(x_1 - \bar{x}_1)^2$
1		
2		
3		
$\Sigma x_1 =$	$\Sigma(x_1 - \bar{x}_1) = 0$	$\Sigma(x_1 - \bar{x}_1)^2 =$

What is n_1?
What is $\bar{x}_1$?
What is $\Sigma(x_1 - \bar{x}_1)^2$?

$n_1 = 3$
$\bar{x}_1 = 2$
$\Sigma(x_1 - \bar{x}_1)^2 = 2$

17.52 *cont'd*
Suppose the 2nd sample is 0, 2, 2, 4:

x_2	$(x_2 - \bar{x}_2)$	$(x_2 - \bar{x}_2)^2$
0		
2		
2		
4		
$\Sigma x_2 =$	$\Sigma(x_2 - \bar{x}_2) = 0$	$\Sigma(x_2 - \bar{x}_2)^2 =$

What is n_2?
What is $\bar{x}_2$?
What is $\Sigma(x_2 - \bar{x}_2)^2$?

$n_2 = 4$
$\bar{x}_2 = 2$
$\Sigma(x_2 - \bar{x}_2)^2 = 8$

         1st sample   2nd sample

$$\therefore s^2 = \frac{\Sigma(x_1 - \bar{x}_1)^2 + \Sigma(x_2 - \bar{x}_2)^2}{n_1 - 1 \quad + \quad n_2 - 1}$$
$$= ?$$

$$\therefore s = ?$$

$$s^2 = \frac{2 + 8}{2 + 3}$$
$$= 2$$

$$s = \sqrt{2}$$

17.53 In the last chapter when we did not know σ_1^2 or σ_2^2 we used

$$z = \frac{\bar{x}_1 - \bar{x}_2}{\sqrt{\dfrac{s_1^2}{n_1} + \dfrac{s_2^2}{n_2}}}$$

for large samples, and kept the two sample variances s_1^2 and s_2^2 separate in estimating σ_1^2 and σ_2^2 respectively. For small samples, we need to use t, and must assume equal variance σ^2 in the underlying populations. (Formally, this assumption should be checked.) Now we must pool the information from the two samples and calculate one value s^2, which =

$$s^2 = \frac{\Sigma(x_1 - \bar{x}_1)^2 + \Sigma(x_2 - \bar{x}_2)^2}{n_1 - 1 + n_2 - 1}$$

$$= \frac{(n_1 - 1)s_1^2 + (n_2 - 1)s_2^2}{n_1 + n_2 - 2}$$

17.54 Having calculated s^2 we use the formula
$t =$

$$t = \frac{\bar{x}_1 - \bar{x}_2}{s\sqrt{\dfrac{1}{n_1} + \dfrac{1}{n_2}}}$$

17.54 *cont'd*

To be precise, if the variances in both samples are not approximately equal we must do something else. The required procedure is a little more complex, however, and so we will not pursue this problem further here.

17.55 f always equals the denominator when s^2 is calculated. Therefore to use t when σ is not known and the sums of squares of the deviations from the means are pooled, $f =$

$$n_1 - 1 + n_2 - 1 = n_1 + n_2 - 2$$

17.56 Here are some fictitious results.
The suggestion is that alcohol slows the reaction time. A very small sample of students was taken, 5 of whom were given a reasonable amount of alcohol and 3 of whom drank fruit juice. As soon as an electric bell rang each was to press a button. The time lapse was recorded electronically.
These are the reaction times:

Fruit juice	Alcohol
10 units	10 units
12 units	12 units
14 units	14 units
	16 units
	18 units

Perform the first step in the significance test.

The Null Hypothesis is that any difference is due only to chance.
The alternative is that alcohol slows the reaction (i.e. increases the reaction time).

17.57 Complete this table and calculate your t value.

	1st sample			2nd sample	
x_1	$x_1 - \bar{x}_1$	$(x_1 - \bar{x}_1)^2$	x_2	$x_2 - \bar{x}_2$	$(x_2 - \bar{x}_2)^2$
10			10		
12			12		
14			14		
			16		
			18		
$\sum x_1 = 0$		$\sum(x_1 - \bar{x}_1)^2 =$	$\sum x_2 = 0$		$\sum(x_2 - \bar{x}_2)^2 =$

17.57   *cont'd*

$\bar{x}_1 =$ $\bar{x}_2 =$
$n_1 =$ $n_2 =$

$s^2 =$

$s =$
$f =$

$$t = \frac{\bar{x}_1 - \bar{x}_2}{s\sqrt{\dfrac{1}{n_1} + \dfrac{1}{n_2}}} =$$

$\bar{x}_1 = 12$ $\bar{x}_2 = 14$
$n_1 = 3$ $n_2 = 5$

$$s^2 = \frac{(4+0+4)+}{6} \frac{(16+4+0+4+16)}{}$$

$= 8$

$s = \sqrt{8}$
$f = 6$ (the denominator)

$$t = \frac{12 - 14}{\sqrt{8}\sqrt{\dfrac{1}{3} + \dfrac{1}{5}}} \approx -1$$

Calculated $t \approx -1$

17.58   The hypothesis in Frame 17.56 is concerned with .... tail(s).

       one

     The significant values (critical values) of t are under the columns headed .... and .... on the row $f =$
Hence significant t values from the t tables on page 279 are ....

       0.10
       0.02, $f = 6$
       1.943 for the 0.05 (5%) level
       3.143 for the 0.01 (1%) level

17.59   The significant value of t is bigger than the calculated value of t. Represent this fact in a sketch.
What is your conclusion?

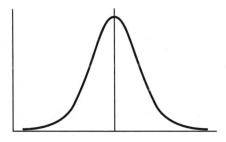

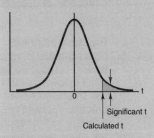

There is no significant difference. Accept the Null Hypothesis. Either alcohol does not slow the reaction time or, if it does, there is insufficient evidence here to show that.

17.60   State the conditions for using a t test.

Random samples.
Quantitative data.
Normal distribution.
n less than 30 and σ unknown.

17.60   *cont'd*

(To repeat, however, even when n is 30 or larger, if σ is unknown, the t test is the strictly correct one, and the z test is only an approximation to it – albeit a good one, especially as n gets larger.)

17.61   The formula for calculating pooled s^2 where σ is unknown is

$$s^2 = \frac{\sum(x_1 - \bar{x}_1)^2 + \sum(x_2 - \bar{x}_2)^2}{n_1 + n_2 - 2}$$

Write this formula without using the means.

$$s^2 = \frac{\sum(x_1{}^2) - \frac{(\sum x_1)^2}{n_1} + \sum(x_2{}^2) - \frac{(\sum x_2)^2}{n_2}}{n_1 + n_2 - 2}$$

Use this result in the example below.

17.62   **Practical example**
In Frames 3.1 and 3.5 we have random samples of birth-weights of children of diabetic and non-diabetic mothers. Are the birth-weights of children of diabetic mothers significantly bigger than those of the control group? You undertook most of the arithmetic in the Practical example at the end of Chapter 7.

For the answer see page 257.

17.63   **Practical example**
This schedule is included as a summary to help you decide the right test to use in the 3 following practical examples which are specially chosen so that you can practise deciding which z or t test to use. Assume all the results in the examples are random and based on normally distributed data.

First you decide whether σ or s is to be used. If σ is unknown the decision about which test to use is based on sample size, but in either case the next decision is whether μ is known (when the test depends on the distribution of the sample mean) or μ is unknown (when the test depends on the distribution of the difference of two sample means).

SUMMARY

Consider the questions in turn and decide on the test depending on the answers.

Is σ known?		Is μ known?
If yes, use z tests		If yes, use $z = \dfrac{\overline{x} - \mu}{\dfrac{\sigma}{\sqrt{n}}}$
		If no, use $z = \dfrac{\overline{x}_1 - \overline{x}_2}{\sigma \sqrt{\dfrac{1}{n_1} + \dfrac{1}{n_2}}}$
If no, z tests may be used in large samples and t tests in small samples	Is $n = 30$ or more for each sample? If yes, z tests may be used as an approximation to the t tests:	If yes, use $z = \dfrac{\overline{x} - \mu}{\dfrac{s}{\sqrt{n}}}$
		If no, use $z = \dfrac{\overline{x}_1 - \overline{x}_2}{\sqrt{\dfrac{s_1^2}{n_1} + \dfrac{s_2^2}{n_2}}}$
	If no, t tests are used:	If yes, use $t = \dfrac{\overline{x} - \mu}{\dfrac{s}{\sqrt{n}}}$ $(f = n - 1)$
		If pairs of differences $(\mu = 0)$, use $t = \dfrac{\overline{x} - 0}{\dfrac{s}{\sqrt{n}}}$ on the differences $(f = n - 1)$ where n is the number of differences
		If μ not known, use $t = \dfrac{\overline{x}_1 - \overline{x}_2}{s \sqrt{\dfrac{1}{n_1} + \dfrac{1}{n_2}}}$ where $s^2 = \dfrac{\Sigma(x - \overline{x}_1)^2 + \Sigma(x - \overline{x}_2)^2}{n_1 + n_2 - 2}$ and $f = n_1 + n_2 - 2$

1. Two students measured the length of the caecum in 25 male and 20 female specimens of a particular animal. They were interested to find out whether the caecal length was significantly different in the two sexes. They calculated the average male caecal length as 14.8 cm and that for females as 13.7 cm.
   What formula would they use to calculate s^2?
   What do the symbols in the formula represent?
   They calculated s^2 correctly to be equal to 0.81.
   What conclusion do they draw? (Answer is on page 257.)

2. Professor X had the idea that people with cancer of the stomach ate more than others. He paired each of his 25 cases of cancer of the stomach with another patient with a different diagnosis but of the same age, sex, race and social class.
   He analysed the average daily intake and found that the mean difference was 180 calories (those with cancer eating more). The standard deviation of the differences was 450 calories.
   What is his conclusion? (Answer is on page 258.)

3. A Secretary for Health wanted to know whether a higher number of car accidents could be related to drivers with increased blood alcohol levels. He took blood samples of 100 randomly selected drivers involved in car accidents and the police chose 100 drivers randomly who had not been involved in an accident. For those involved in accidents the mean alcohol level was 2.42 units with a variance of 0.39. For the control group the mean was 2.24 units with a variance of 0.25.
   What conclusion would the Secretary draw?
   (Answer is on page 259.)

18. Testing for real correlation

INTRODUCTION

In Chapters 8 and 9 we learnt about correlation and how to calculate the correlation coefficients r and ρ. By chance a positive or negative – i.e. non-zero – value of the coefficient would almost always be calculated, even when in fact there existed no real correlation. Indeed it is exceedingly rare to obtain the exact result r or $\rho = 0$. This chapter shows you how to decide whether a particular value for r or ρ is likely to be due to significant correlation or chance variation from 0.

18.1	What does $1 - \dfrac{6\sum d^2}{n(n^2 - 1)}$ equal?	ρ, Spearman's coefficient of rank correlation
18.2	What is 'd' in the above equation?	The difference between the rankings of a pair of variables
18.3	What is the name of the other correlation coefficient you have met?	Pearson's product-moment correlation coefficient, r
18.4	Suppose that you wished to decide whether a value of $r = +0.1$ represented real correlation or just a chance variation from $r = 0$. What would your Null Hypothesis be?	That the variation from 0 was entirely due to chance
18.5	If you were interested in detecting real negative correlation this would involve a .... tailed test. Where no sign is specified a .... tailed test is required. The last frame required a .... tailed test.	one two two
18.6	To test your Null Hypothesis you use $t = \dfrac{r\sqrt{n-2}}{\sqrt{1-r^2}}$ What does n represent?	The number of pairs of results

| 18.7 | To use this formula r and ρ are interchangeable. Hence, what is the formula for testing whether a value of ρ represents real correlation? | $t = \dfrac{\rho \sqrt{n-2}}{\sqrt{1-\rho^2}}$ |

| 18.8 | In this particular t test,
$f = n - 2$.
What does f represent? | f is the number of degrees of freedom. |

| 18.9 | Suppose the correlation coefficient, $+0.1$, was calculated from 11 pairs of results.
Then $f = ?$ | $f = n - 2 = 9$ |

| 18.10 | We have:
$r = +0.1$
$n = 11$
So, $t = ?$

(Substitute in the formula in Frame 18.6.) | $t = \dfrac{+0.1 \sqrt{9}}{\sqrt{1-0.01}}$

$= \dfrac{+0.3}{\sqrt{0.99}} \simeq +0.3$ |

| 18.11 | The calculated value of $t = +0.3$.
What does f equal again?
What are the corresponding significant t values (critical values) in the 't' tables? (Two-tailed test.) | $f = 9$
$t = 2.262$ at the 0.05 (5%) level
$t = 3.250$ at the 0.01 (1%) level |

| 18.12 | Is the calculated t bigger than the significant (critical) t? | No. $+0.3$ is smaller than both 2.262 and 3.250. |

| 18.13 | Do you reject the Null Hypothesis? | No |

| 18.14 | Do you conclude that the correlation coefficient $+0.1$ here represents only chance variation from 0? | Yes, or that there is insufficient evidence to suggest otherwise |

| 18.15 | Suppose that height and weight in a group of people are correlated, with $r = +0.6$. You wish to test whether this represents real +ve correlation.

Then this is a .... tailed test. | one |

18.16 There are 27 members of the group measured, so

$$t = \frac{r\sqrt{n-2}}{\sqrt{1-r^2}} = ?$$

$f = ?$

$$t = \frac{0.6\sqrt{25}}{\sqrt{1-0.36}} = \frac{3}{0.8}$$

$$= 3.75$$

$f = 25$

18.17 The calculated value of $t = 3.75$, and the significant (critical) value of $t = ?$ (From the tables.)

1.708 at the 0.05 (5%) level
2.485 at the 0.01 (1%) level

18.18 What is your conclusion?

There is very strong evidence that there is real +ve correlation between height and weight in the group of people.

18.19 Had only 6 members of the group been present, what would your conclusion have been, assuming the same correlation coefficient?

We now have:

$$t = \frac{0.6\sqrt{4}}{\sqrt{1-0.36}} = \frac{1.2}{0.8} = 1.5$$

and $f = 4$.

This result needs to be compared with the following significant (critical) values of t:
2.132 at the 0.05 (5%) level
3.747 at the 0.01 (1%) level

The conclusion would now be that the correlation was not real, or that there was insufficient evidence to suggest otherwise.

18.20 **Practical example**
What conclusion do you draw about your values for r and ρ calculated at the end of Chapter 9? Do the data represent real correlation? (Answer is on page 260.)

SUMMARY

The formula used for testing the Null Hypothesis that there is no real correlation is

$$t = \frac{r\sqrt{n-2}}{\sqrt{1-r^2}}$$ (for Pearson's product-moment correlation coefficient), or

$$\frac{\rho\sqrt{n-2}}{\sqrt{1-\rho^2}}$$ (for Spearman's rank correlation coefficient), where $f = n - 2$.

Discussion about which tests to use if your data are quantitative

Some readers may feel that although they can understand the frames individually they would still be confused about which tests they should use if faced with research data to analyse from scratch. This short discussion is intended for people who feel that they are in that position.

In the past some medical students have undertaken small holiday research projects. Here are four modified examples. See whether you would now be able to perform the necessary tests. Remember, from the statistical point of view, it is as important to realise your limitations as to know which tests are within your capabilities. You are not yet in a position to analyse all sets of data!

Project 1
Three students measured the X-ray width of the 1st thoracic vertebra of 3 different groups of people. There were 100 in each group. The students wished to know whether the 3 groups differed. Are you able to perform the applicable calculation?

No, except to compare the groups two at a time using

$$z = \frac{\bar{x}_1 - \bar{x}_2}{\sqrt{\dfrac{s_1^2}{n_1} + \dfrac{s_2^2}{n_2}}}$$

Three groups are properly compared together using the 'analysis of variance' technique which you do not know from this learning programme. (Incidentally, there was no difference found.)

Project 2
A student measured:

- (x) the average rise in the height of the diaphragm relative to the ribs, and
- (y) the increase in the area of the heart and pedicle.

Project 2 *cont'd*
He had 60 of each measurement on a group of 60 X-rays. He wanted to know whether the variable (X) was associated with (Y).
If he had given you his results could you have given him the answer?

Describe how you would have answered his problem.

Yes, we hope so.

You should have used Pearson's product-moment correlation coefficient, given by:

$$r = \frac{\Sigma(xy) - \frac{(\Sigma x)(\Sigma y)}{n}}{\sqrt{\Sigma(x^2) - \frac{(\Sigma x)^2}{n}} \ \sqrt{\Sigma(y^2) - \frac{(\Sigma y)^2}{n}}}$$

to test whether the calculated correlation coefficient was significantly different from zero and you should have computed the test statistic t, given by:

$$t = \frac{r\sqrt{n-2}}{\sqrt{1 - r^2}}$$

The appropriate test is two-tailed, on $f = 58$ degrees of freedom.

(An association – a significant correlation – was found.)

Project 3
Another student wanted to compare the number of Kalanga tribesmen with a whorl on the fingerprint of their right thumb, with the number in the Nanjanga tribe.
Could you work this out, given the data?

No, those with whorls were counted, leading to qualitative data.
This is the subject of the next chapter.
(He found no difference.)

Project 4
Two exchange students from other universities measured the heights of (1) 35 eleven-year-old schoolboys with goitres and (2) 30 eleven-year-old schoolboys without goitres at a local mission school. They wanted to know

$$z = \frac{\bar{x}_1 - \bar{x}_2}{\sqrt{\frac{s_1^2}{n_1} + \frac{s_2^2}{n_2}}}$$

Project 4 *cont'd*
whether the boys without goitres were bigger than those with. What formula would you use?
Is this a one- or two-tailed test?

(This approximate result is acceptable because the size of both samples is at least 30. However, the strictly correct approach if the population variances are equal ($\sigma_1^2 = \sigma_2^2$) is to use

$$t = \frac{\bar{x}_1 - \bar{x}_2}{s\sqrt{\dfrac{1}{n_1} + \dfrac{1}{n_2}}},$$

where

$$s^2 = \frac{(n_1 - 1)s_1^2 + (n_2 - 1)s_2^2}{n_1 + n_2 - 2},$$

and it would certainly be appropriate to use this.)

One-tailed. (They found that boys without goitres were not significantly bigger.)

CONCLUSION

Although after completing this programme so far you are still limited in your knowledge of actual tests which are in use, the basic ideas are always those that you now know.

You should now always be able to understand what statistical tests are about and what your statistical conclusions mean.

19. Simple linear regression

INTRODUCTION

We have seen how correlation coefficients can give us information on the degree of linear association between a pair of variables. However, they tell us nothing about the slope of any line that might provide a reasonable description of the bivariate data (i.e. information on two variables). That is a key feature of simple linear regression. A regression analysis is appropriate when we have a pair of variables which are linearly related. A line is fitted to the data and can be used to predict values of the variable of interest, for given values of what is called the independent variable.

19.1	What does correlation measure?	Linear association
19.2	What is the possible range of values for a correlation coefficient?	-1 to $+1$
19.3	What does a correlation coefficient of 0 mean?	No linear association between a pair of variables. Remember, this is not the same as no association at all. There may be a strong curvilinear association between a pair of variables, yet the coefficient of correlation between them may be zero, or very nearly so.
19.4	What does a correlation coefficient of $+1$ mean?	Perfect positive linear association between a pair of variables
19.5	What does the correlation coefficient of $+1$ tell you about the slope of the line passing through the data points?	Nothing
19.6	What does any correlation coefficient tell you about the slope of a line fitted to the data?	Nothing

19.7   What is a statistic?

It is some function of sample data values.

19.8   Do you know what the statistic is called that tells you something about the slope of the line, in a linear relationship between a pair of variables?
(*Hint*: Correlation is about linear association between a pair of variables, and the correlation coefficient tells us something about the degree of association. Regression is about a linear relationship between a pair of variables and the .... coefficient tells us something about the slope of the line.)

The regression coefficient

◦ regression

19.9   Look at the diagram below. Why is it easy to decide which is the 'best' straight line to fit to the points plotted there?

All the 4 points lie exactly on the straight line, so there is no question of any alternative possibilities.

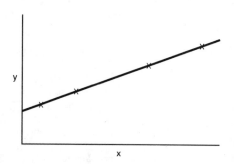

19.10 Look at the diagram below. Why is it now not so easy to decide which is the 'best' (in some sense) straight line to fit to the plotted points?

The 4 points no longer lie exactly on any straight line. It is no longer clear which straight line fits the points best – nor, indeed, what 'best' means in this context. A possible line has been drawn in the diagram, but it is not the only possible line.

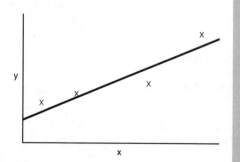

19.11　In the diagram below, what is the slope of the line?

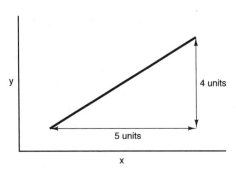

The slope is $\frac{4}{5}$, or 0.8.

19.12　In the diagram below, what is the slope of the line?

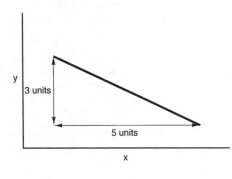

The slope is $\frac{-3}{5}$, or −0.6.

19.13　In Frames 19.11 and 19.12 what do the signs and magnitudes of the slopes indicate?

The sign indicates the *direction* of the line. A positive slope indicates a line going uphill (from left to right), whereas a negative sign indicates a line going downhill (from left to right). The magnitude of the slope indicates how *steep* the line is.

19.14　In the diagram below, what is the slope of the line?

The slope is $\dfrac{5}{\frac{1}{2}} = 10$.

19.14   *cont'd*

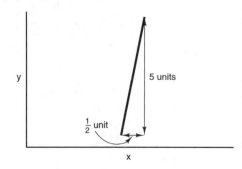

19.15   What is the range of possible values of the slope of a line?

Very steep uphill lines have a very large positive value for the slope. Very steep downhill lines have a very large negative value for the slope. Lines with very shallow gradient (i.e. almost horizontal) have a slope close to zero (just positive, or just negative, depending on whether the line is gently sloping uphill or downhill). So slopes can take all possible values from $-\infty$ (minus infinity), through 0, to $+\infty$ (plus infinity).

19.16   What sort of line has zero slope?

A horizontal line

19.17   What sort of line has infinitely large (positive or negative) slope?

A vertical line

19.18   What range of values can a correlation coefficient take?

From -1 to 1

19.19   What is the name of the coefficient that measures the slope of a fitted straight line?

A regression coefficient

19.20   What range of values can a regression coefficient take?

The same as the slope: from $-\infty$ to $+\infty$

19.21 In a situation like the one depicted in Frame 19.10 you might think that the best way to fit a line to the points is simply to do so by eye and to draw it in by hand. Why would this not be a good way of doing it, in general?

This approach is subjective rather than objective. Given the same set of points to be fitted, different individuals are likely to fit different lines. Even the same individual is likely to fit slightly different lines to the same set of points, if doing so repeatedly.

19.22 Suppose a line has been fitted to a set of points by eye. What is the name given to the slope?

The regression coefficient

19.23 With the line having been fitted subjectively, by eye, what formal inferences can be drawn about the magnitude of the regression coefficient?

None at all. Because of the subjective nature of the fitting, there is no reference point with which to compare the observed value of the regression coefficient.

19.24 Clearly, we cannot progress very far like this. We need an objective way of fitting lines to observed points (bivariate data). We need to have a criterion for deciding what is the *line of best fit* to a set of data.

19.25 We need to arrange that the fitted line is in some sense as close as possible to all the observed points.

19.26 What is a way of transforming positive and negative values so that they all end up positive? (*Hint*: Remember what we did to construct the formula for the variance.)

Square all the numbers. The squares of both positive numbers and negative numbers are positive.

19.27 Consider again the diagram in Frame 19.10. Perpendicular distances of the points from a fitted line have been marked on the diagram.

19.27   *cont'd*

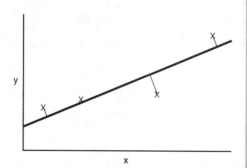

Bearing in mind what we have said in Frame 19.26, what might be a reasonable approach to fitting a line to the points?

A possible approach would be to choose the line which minimises the sum of the squares of the perpendicular distances of the points from the line.

19.28   In fact, this is not quite what we do, but we have now established a useful principle which can be easily amended to provide what we require. When we compute a correlation coefficient between two variables, which of the variables is more important?

Neither. The variables have equal status. In computing a correlation coefficient we are simply interested in quantifying the degree of linear association between a pair of variables.

19.29   When we fit a straight line – a regression line – to a set of data (i.e. we carry out a simple linear regression analysis – a multiple linear regression analysis occurs when we have more than two variables of interest) we are often interested in using the fitted line to predict a value of one variable, say Y, given a value of another variable, say X. So now, the variables do not have equal status. In the above we would call X the independent variable, or regressor variable, and Y the dependent variable. We think of the X values as being fixed. Can you think of some examples where we may wish to predict the value of one variable, given the value of another?

Clearly there are many possible examples. Some follow:
1. Prediction of weight, given height, for a normal healthy person (males and females separately).
2. Prediction of forced expiratory volume, given a fixed length of time on an exercise bike, for a normal, healthy person (males and females separately).
3. Prediction of heart rate given a fixed time

| 19.29 | *cont'd* | of running on a treadmill, for normal healthy people (males and females separately). |

19.30   Note that it is quite clear in two of the examples quoted (2 and 3) which one of the variables can be fixed, allowing the other to vary. (In example 2, it is the length of time on the exercise bike that can be fixed. In example 3 it is the time of running on the treadmill.) The fixed variable is the independent, or regressor variable. (This is quite typical of experimental situations.) The situation is not quite so clear-cut in example 1, though it is clear that we would be interested in predicting weight from height, rather than the other way round, when, for example, investigating the health of the nation, eating habits, propensity for obesity etc.

19.31   All this leads us to the concept of a regression line of Y on X. In this case, which is the independent (regressor) variable, and which is the dependent variable?

X is the independent (regressor) variable; Y is the dependent variable.

19.32   For a pair of variables X, Y, there is also another regression line – that of X on Y. (But note that it would rarely make sense to consider both the line of Y on X and the line of X on Y for the same set of data.) Now which is the independent (regressor) variable, and which is the dependent variable?

Y is the independent (regressor) variable; X is the dependent variable.

19.33   We usually work with the regression line of Y on X. Let us consider how to fit such a line to a set of data. Look again at the diagram depicted in Frame 19.10. Vertical distances (i.e. parallel to the y axis) of points from the line have now been drawn in.

19.33　*cont'd*

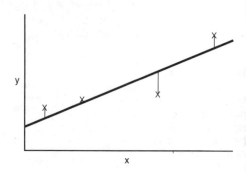

Bearing in mind what we have discussed so far, can you suggest how the best fitting line of *Y* on *X* is chosen?

The line is chosen so that the sum of the squares of the vertical distances of the points from the line is minimised. It is clear that this is the appropriate direction in which to consider the differences once we realise that it is the *X* values which are fixed.

19.34　The method used in Frame 19.33 for fitting the line to the data is called the *principle of least squares* (for an obvious reason).

19.35　What do you think the full name of the fitted line for *Y* on *X* is?

It is the least squares line of regression of *Y* on *X*.

19.36　In fitting the regression line of *Y* on *X* we are seeking a line of the form $y = \alpha + \beta x$, where α and β are to be estimated from the data by quantities a and b, respectively, which we will meet further on. α and β are called parameters. α is the value of the y-intercept (i.e. the value of y at the point where the line crosses the y axis). β corresponds to the slope of the line. What else do we call it?

The regression coefficient

19.37　The sum of squares of the vertical distances from the points (x, y) to the

19.37 *cont'd*
fitted line is expressed as a function of x and y, and mathematics is used to find those values of a and b, in terms of x and y, which minimise the sum of squares. This is fortunate, because it simply leads us to formulae for a and b, in terms of the observed x and y values.

19.38 We will not go through the details of the calculations here.
The formula for b, the least squares estimate of β, is

$$b = \frac{\sum(x - \bar{x})(y - \bar{y})}{\sum(x - \bar{x})^2}$$

For computational purposes this can be expressed as

$$\frac{\sum(xy) - \dfrac{(\sum x)(\sum y)}{n}}{\sum(x^2) - \dfrac{(\sum x)^2}{n}}$$

19.39 Once we have calculated the value of b from the data, the value of a, the least squares estimate of α, can be calculated from the formula

$$a = \bar{y} - b\bar{x}$$

19.40 The fitted line (the least squares regression line of Y on X) is then given by

$$y = a + bx$$

19.41 If $a = \bar{y} - b\bar{x}$ and $y = a + bx$, derive an equation for $(y - \bar{y})$ not involving a.

Substituting $a = \bar{y} - b\bar{x}$ into the second equation we have $y = \bar{y} - b\bar{x} + bx$. This in itself is a useful equation, because it shows how to predict a value of y, given a value of x. However, carrying on, and subtracting $\bar{y}$ from each side of the equation, we have:
$(y - \bar{y}) = b(x - \bar{x})$.

19.42 Given the form of the regression line just derived in Frame 19.41, what particular point of interest does the regression line necessarily pass through?

The mean of the array of observed points, i.e. the point $(\bar{x}, \bar{y})$. (This is simply the point on the line when x takes the value $\bar{x}$.)

19.43 Describe the fitted regression line of Y on X.

It is the line with slope b passing through the mean of the array of observed points, $(\bar{x}, \bar{y})$. This line minimises the sum of squared vertical distances of the observed points from the fitted line.

19.44 Let us now consider an example. Research on digestion requires accurate measurements of blood flow through the lining of the stomach. A method for obtaining such measurements is to inject mildly radioactive microscopic spheres into the bloodstream. The spheres lodge in tiny blood vessels at a rate proportional to blood flow. Their radioactivity allows blood flow to be measured from outside the body. In an experiment, researchers compared the blood flow rate (BFR) measured by the use of microspheres with simultaneous measurements of actual blood flow taken using a catheter inserted into a vein. The results were as follows:

Measurement	Sphere BFR (x) (ml/min)	Catheter BFR (y) (ml/min)
1	4.0	3.3
2	4.7	8.3
3	6.3	4.5
4	8.2	9.3
5	12.0	10.7
6	15.9	16.4
7	17.4	15.4
8	18.1	17.6
9	20.2	21.0
10	23.9	21.7

Source: 'Measurements of gastric blood flow with radioactive microspheres', L. H. Archibald, F. G. Moody and M. J. Simons, *Applied Physiology* 38 (1975), pp. 1051–6.

19.45 In the example in Frame 19.44, the sphere BFR is being used as a proxy for the catheter (true) BFR. On another occasion it might be hoped to measure just the sphere BFR (having calibrated it against catheter BFR in the experiment). In the regression analysis that will follow, which will therefore be the dependent variable and which the independent (regressor) variable?

The catheter BFR will be the dependent variable (Y) and the sphere BFR will be the independent (regressor) variable (X). (The practical interest here is being able to predict the catheter BFR (the true rate) from the more easily measured sphere BFR, so that the sphere BFR can be used as a proxy measure in future.)

19.46 Plot catheter BFR against sphere BFR in a scatter diagram.

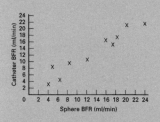

19.47 Does inspection of the data lead you to believe that a linear regression analysis will be appropriate here?

Yes. There appears to be a strong linear relationship, and no problems with unequal variance.

19.48 What type of relationship between y and x should we fit to the data?

$y = \alpha + \beta x$. In fact, what we fit is $y = a + bx$, where a and b are estimates of α and β respectively. More specifically, the model is $y = \alpha + \beta x + \varepsilon$, where the error term ε associated with the point (x, y) is normally distributed with mean 0 and variance σ^2 (and it then follows that when X is equal to x, the mean of Y is equal to $\alpha + \beta x$).

19.49 Compute the regression coefficient for this set of data (as introduced in Frame 19.44).

x	y	x^2	xy	y^2
4.0	3.3	16.00	13.20	10.89
4.7	8.3	22.09	39.01	68.89
6.3	4.5	39.69	28.35	20.25
8.2	9.3	67.24	76.26	86.49
12.0	10.7	144.00	128.40	114.49
15.9	16.4	252.81	260.76	268.96
17.4	15.4	302.76	267.96	237.16
18.1	17.6	327.61	318.56	309.76
20.2	21.0	408.04	424.20	441.00
23.9	21.7	571.21	518.63	470.89

$\Sigma x = 130.7$
$\Sigma y = 128.2$
$\Sigma(x^2) = 2151.45$
$\Sigma(xy) = 2075.33$

$$b = \frac{\Sigma(xy) - \dfrac{(\Sigma x)(\Sigma y)}{n}}{\Sigma(x^2) - \dfrac{(\Sigma x)^2}{n}}$$

$$= \frac{2075.33 - \dfrac{(130.7) \times (128.2)}{10}}{2151.45 - \dfrac{(130.7)^2}{10}}$$

$$= \frac{399.756}{443.201} = 0.9020$$

19.50 Compute the y-intercept a for the same set of data.

$\bar{y} = \dfrac{128.2}{10} = 12.82$

$\bar{x} = \dfrac{130.7}{10} = 13.07$

So $a = \bar{y} - b\bar{x}$

$= 12.82 - (0.9020) \times (13.07)$

$= 1.0309$

19.51 What is the least squares regression line of Y on X for the data of Frame 19.44?

$y = 1.0309 + 0.9020x$

19.52 Plot the fitted regression line of Y on X on the scatter diagram of y and x values.

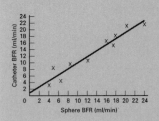

19.53	Having fitted a regression line to a set of data, the question is often asked, 'Is the regression significant?' This is, in fact, not a very clearly expressed question. But what do you think it means, in more precise terms?	What the question is really asking, although it has not been very carefully expressed, is: 'Is the estimated regression coefficient, b, significantly different from zero?'
19.54	A more precise question would therefore be 'Is the regression coefficient, β, different from zero?' What does this mean, in practical terms?	It means 'Has the fitted line got a slope which is significantly different from zero?', or, in other words, 'Is the fitted line significantly different from a horizontal line?' (which corresponds to there being no evidence of a linear relationship between X and Y).
19.55	Are we equipped to answer this question, from what we know already?	No. We do not know what to compare the estimated value of β, b, with in order to be able to give an answer.
19.56	What do we need to know to be able to answer the question in Frame 19.53? (This is a question about β, estimated by b.)	We need to know what the standard error of b is.
19.57	In order to see what the standard error of b is we need first of all to consider what the underlying model for the regression line is.	
19.58	What is a model in the context of modelling a set of data?	It is a relationship expressed in terms of parameters to be estimated from the data.
19.59	In a simple linear regression analysis of Y on X what form of relationship are we aiming to fit to the data?	$y = \alpha + \beta x$

19.60 As we have seen, in general the regression line does not fit all the observed points exactly. In other words, there is a random error associated with each point (corresponding to the vertical distance to the line in the diagram in Frame 19.33). Suppose the error is represented by ε, for point (x, y). How can the model be expressed for the point (x, y)?

$y = \alpha + \beta x + \varepsilon$
This makes it clear that for each value x of X it is the means of Y that we think of as being linearly related to the x values. There is variation about the line for the individual observed values y.

19.61 In order to fully specify the model certain assumptions are required concerning the error term. It is assumed that the ε are mutually independent and that they each have a normal distribution with mean 0 and variance σ^2, say. We will return to the implications of these assumptions a little later, but we can now see what the standard error of b is.

19.62 Now that we have seen what σ^2 is, we can state that the variance of b is given by

$$\frac{\sigma^2}{\Sigma(x - \bar{x})^2}$$

Note that how precise b is as an estimate of β, the slope of the regression line, depends on how much scatter about the line there is of the observed points.

19.63 In that case, what is the standard error of b?

The standard error is the square root of the variance,

i.e. $\dfrac{\sigma}{\sqrt{\Sigma(x - \bar{x})^2}}$

This provides a basis for a confidence interval for the slope, which takes the form

$$b \pm z \times \frac{\sigma}{\sqrt{\Sigma(x - \bar{x})^2}}$$

if σ is known, or

$$b \pm t \times \frac{\text{Estimate of } \sigma}{\sqrt{(x - \bar{x})^2}}$$

19.63 *cont'd*

if σ is not known (see Frames 19.66 and 19.67 for the estimate of σ). z and t are the appropriate values (depending on whether the interval is 95%, 90% etc.) from the normal and Student's t distributions respectively.

19.64 Do we know σ^2?

No

19.65 So what do we have to do?

Estimate it from the data

19.66 Now we have established the principles of what we have to do we will simply proceed to see how we test b for significance, rather than working through the detailed algebra. We need the following expressions:

$$(A) = \text{(sum of } x^2) - \frac{\text{(sum of } x)^2}{n}$$

$$= \Sigma(x^2) - \frac{(\Sigma x)^2}{n}$$

$$(B) = \text{(sum of } y^2) - \frac{\text{(sum of } y)^2}{n}$$

$$= \Sigma(y^2) - \frac{(\Sigma y)^2}{n}$$

$$(C) = \text{(sum of } xy) - \frac{\text{(sum of } x)\text{(sum of } y)}{n}$$

$$= \Sigma(xy) - \frac{(\Sigma x)(\Sigma y)}{n}$$

Next we compute (D), where

$$(D) = \frac{1}{(n-2)}\left[(B) - \frac{(C)^2}{(A)}\right]$$

19.67 This last step is the one where we are estimating σ^2 – the estimate is given by (D). Looking at the form of the formula, and remembering the formula for a sample variance, for example, how many degrees of freedom, f, do you think the estimate is based on?

$f = n - 2$
Note that what this formula corresponds to is the sum of squares of differences between observed and predicted (from the linear relationship) values, divided by the number of degrees of freedom.

19.68 Since we are having to estimate the value of σ^2, what type of test do you think we will end up carrying out for the significance of b?

A t test

19.69 We now compute (E), given by

$$(E) = \sqrt{\frac{(D)}{(A)}}$$

Do you recognise how the form of this matches Frame 19.62?

We hope so!

19.70 We have finally got all that we require, and can now proceed to compute the test statistic! It is given by

$$(T) = \frac{b}{(E)}$$

What form does this have?

$$\frac{b}{\text{standard error of } b},$$

i.e. the same format as other test statistics that we have seen.

19.71 What set of tables will you compare the computed value with?

Tables of the t distribution

19.72 Under what number of degrees of freedom, f, will you look up the value?

$f = n - 2$

19.73 We now have all that we require to be able to test whether the slope of the fitted regression line is significantly different from zero. What else might we like to know about the line?

Whether or not it passes through the origin

19.74 Which parameter in the model will give us information about whether the line passes through the origin or not?

α, the y-intercept

19.75 What test do we need to carry out?

A test of whether α is different from zero, by determining whether its estimate, a, is significantly different from zero

19.76   If it turns out that the fitted y-intercept is not significantly different from zero, can we infer that a line through the origin would describe the data well?

> Yes, as long as we have assured ourselves that a straight line is appropriate for the data

19.77   What do you think the format of the test statistic for α is?

$$\frac{a}{\text{standard error of } a}$$

19.78   In order to carry out the test for α we need to compute the expression (G), where

$$(G) = \sqrt{(D)\left[\frac{1}{n} + \frac{(\overline{x})^2}{(A)}\right]}$$

Then the appropriate test statistic is given by (V), where

$$(V) = \frac{a}{(G)}$$

The computed value is compared with tabulated values of the t distribution with $(n - 2)$ degrees of freedom.

19.79   Refer back to Frames 19.49 and 19.66. For the data of Frame 19.44 compute the values (A), (B), (C) and hence (D).

$$(A) = \Sigma(x^2) - \frac{(\Sigma x)^2}{n}$$

$$= 443.201,$$
from Frame 19.49

$$(B) = \Sigma(y^2) - \frac{(\Sigma y)^2}{n}$$

$$= 2028.78 - \frac{(128.2)^2}{10}$$

$$= 385.256$$

$$(C) = \Sigma(xy) - \frac{(\Sigma x)(\Sigma y)}{n}$$

$$= 399.756,$$
from Frame 19.49
Then

$$(D) = \frac{1}{(n-2)}\left[(B) - \frac{(C)^2}{(A)}\right]$$

$$= \frac{1}{8}\left[385.256 - \frac{(399.756)^2}{443.201}\right]$$

$$= 3.0858$$

19.80 Referring now to Frame 19.69, compute the value of (E) where $(E) = \sqrt{\dfrac{(D)}{(A)}}$	$(E) = \sqrt{\dfrac{3.0858}{443.201}}$ $= \sqrt{0.006963}$ $= 0.0834$
19.81 What is this quantity that we have just computed?	It is the standard error of b.
19.82 If we want to carry out a test of whether the fitted regression coefficient is significantly different from zero, what is the form of the test statistic?	$\dfrac{b}{\text{standard error of } b}$
19.83 Compute the test statistic referred to in Frame 19.82.	It is $\dfrac{0.9020}{0.0834}$, i.e. 10.82.
19.84 What tabulated values is this statistic to be compared with?	Those of a t distribution with 8 degrees of freedom
19.85 We are simply interested in testing for a difference from zero. No direction of the difference is specified. What are the significant values (critical values) of t at the 0.05 (5%) and 0.01 (1%) levels?	They are: $t = 2.306$ (0.05 level) $t = 3.355$ (0.01 level)
19.86 What is the outcome?	The calculated test statistic is much larger in magnitude than either of these values. Hence $p < 0.01$. In fact, it is also true that $p < 0.001$, so the result is significant at the 0.001 (0.1%) level – we say that the result is very highly significant.
19.87 What other test is of interest for these data?	A test of whether the fitted y-intercept is significantly different from zero This is particularly relevant for the data in question since it is not

| 19.87 | *cont'd* | unreasonable to suppose that catheter BFR might be proportional to sphere BFR. |

19.88 Referring to Frame 19.78 carry out the test for the *y*-intercept.

We require (G), where

$$(G) = \sqrt{(D) \left[\frac{1}{n} + \frac{(\bar{x})^2}{(A)} \right]}$$

Now, $\bar{x} = 13.07$, so

$$(G) = \sqrt{3.0858 \left[\frac{1}{10} + \frac{(13.07)^2}{443.201} \right]}$$

$$= \sqrt{1.4980}$$

$$= 1.2239$$

The test statistic is

$$(V) = \frac{a}{(G)} = \frac{1.0309}{1.2239}$$

$$= 0.84$$

This is compared with tabulated values of the *t* distribution with 8 degrees of freedom corresponding to a two-tailed test (see Frame 19.85). The result is not significant at the 5% level, so the fitted *y*-intercept is not significantly different from zero at the 5% significance level ($p > 0.05$).

19.89 Might a line of proportionality between *Y* and *X* (i.e. a straight line of the form $y = \beta x$, so passing through the origin) be a reasonable model for the data?

According to the result in Frame 19.88 it might be.

19.90 Sometimes we may have two independent sets of data and we may be interested in comparing the two regression lines of *Y* on *X* which are fitted separately to those two sets of data. In particular we may be interested in comparing the regression coefficients,

We are interested in the difference between two slopes, $\beta_1 - \beta_2$, say. This difference is estimated by $b_1 - b_2$. This quantity then needs to be divided by its standard error. So we end

19.90 *cont'd*
or the slopes, for the two lines. In principle, what form do you think an appropriate test would take?

up with a test statistic of familiar form, namely

$$\frac{b_1 - b_2}{\text{standard error of } (b_1 - b_2)}.$$

This is then compared with the appropriate distribution.

19.91 We would then look up the computed value of the test statistic in the tables of which distribution?

t distribution

19.92 We have seen already that the test for a simple regression coefficient is based on $n - 2$ degrees of freedom, where n is the number of pairs of points. We are now concerned with the comparison of a regression coefficient derived from a set of n_1 points with a regression coefficient derived from a set of n_2 points. What do you think is the number of degrees of freedom associated with the test?

It is
$(n_1 - 2) + (n_2 - 2)$
$= (n_1 + n_2 - 4)$.

19.93 We have now established the principle for comparing the regression coefficients from two different lines. So as not to lead you into extensive algebra, however, we will not proceed to the detailed test itself. If you need this, consult a standard textbook on elementary or intermediate statistics.

19.94 We now return briefly to the assumptions underlying the model for a linear regression analysis, and look at the implications of those for the analysis. What is the linear regression model for Y on X, for the point (x, y)?

$y = \alpha + \beta x + \varepsilon$

19.95 What assumptions are made about ε?

The ε values are independently distributed and follow normal distributions with mean 0 and variance σ^2.

19.96 This is what the assumptions mean diagrammatically:

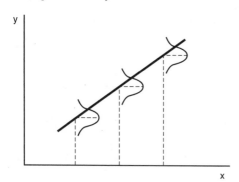

This means that for each of the x values we assume that the corresponding population of y values is symmetrically (normally) distributed about the line. So the actual value y of Y that we observe, for a given value x of X, is more likely to lie close to the line than further away from it, and is equally likely to be above or below the line. The point here is that we do not expect the fitted line to pass exactly through all the observed points. The regression analysis will be most effective if these distributions only have a narrow spread about the line.

19.97 The distributional part of the assumption should be checked by examining residuals (observed minus expected values, from fitting the straight-line model) and seeing whether they are normally distributed.

19.98 One of the assumptions concerns the need for constant variance, or homoscedasticity. Do you know what the word is to describe the situation when there is not constant variance?

It is 'heteroscedasticity'.

19.99 Draw a diagram of what you would expect a set of observations to look like if a linear regression model is appropriate.

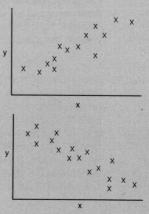

19.100 Can you draw a diagram to indicate what a set of observations might look like if there is non-constant variance in the y values (typically, variance increasing with the x values)?

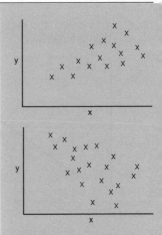

Again, the residuals from fitting the model should be checked for constant variance, though, as in the diagram you have drawn, you may be able to detect a problem of non-constant variance just by looking at the (x, y) values. The moral really is to look at the data before you fit the regression model, and look at the data (residuals) again after fitting the model to the data.

19.101 If either the normality assumption or the constant variance assumption fails – or both do – it is worth trying to transform the data to see if that will improve matters. We will not go into transformations in depth here, but simply note that it is often helpful to try working with log y rather than y, when the assumptions fail.

19.102 Some form of model underlies most statistical analyses. All models are based on assumptions. When the assumptions are not satisfied by the data there are in general two possible courses of action. One is to try transforming the data. Another is to have recourse to nonparametric methods of statistics. They are the subject of Chapter 21.

SUMMARY

Some form of model underlies most statistical analyses.

The model for an observation (x, y) in a simple linear regression analysis takes the form $y = \alpha + \beta x + \varepsilon$ where α and β are constants and ε is an error term.

This is the simple linear regression line of Y on X. There is a corresponding line of X on Y.

In the line of Y on X, Y is the dependent variable and X is the independent, or regressor, variable.

Any model has assumptions underlying it. In the case of the linear regression model the assumptions are that the error terms ε are distributed with zero mean and constant variance. The constant variance criterion is called homoscedasticity. Departure from this is called heteroscedasticity. β is the regression coefficient and defines the slope of the regression line. α determines the y-intercept of the regression line.

A formal test can be carried out in a regression analysis to determine whether the fitted regression coefficient is different from zero. The test reduces to a Student's t test.

Similarly a formal test can be carried out to determine whether the fitted y-intercept is different from zero. This also reduces to a Student's t test. It is relevant to carry out this test when deciding whether a straight line through the origin is appropriate for the data.

When regression lines are fitted to two different data sets it is possible to compare the fitted regression coefficients by means of a formal statistical test. Once again, this reduces to a Student's t test.

20. Simple tests with χ^2

INTRODUCTION

Most tests involving qualitative data depend on χ^2.

20.1	z, t and r are all calculated from qualitative/quantitative data.	quantitative
20.2	What is the distinction between qualitative and quantitative data?	Qualitative data are counted. Quantitative data are measured.
20.3	χ is the Greek letter 'chi', pronounced 'ki' (as in 'kite'). χ^2 tests are called .... tests.	chi-squared
20.4	χ^2 depends on f, like .... (Symbol)	t
20.5	What does f represent?	The number of degrees of freedom
20.6	Qualitative data are usually counted into groups or categories. An example is blood groups. The Null Hypothesis says that any variation between the observed numbers in the groups and what you would expect is due to what?	*Chance* variation only
20.7	If there is a significant difference the variation is .... than is expected by chance and this suggests that some other factor is involved.	more
20.8	As with z and t, if the calculated value of χ^2 is bigger than the significant (critical) value (at the chosen significance level) you accept/reject the Null Hypothesis.	If χ^2 is bigger, p is smaller and the Null Hypothesis is rejected.

20.9 Unlike the z and t tables, the χ^2 tables in this book are used directly in one-/two-tailed tests? (But remember to check exactly what is being presented in any other tables that you may use.)

one-tailed

20.10 Look at the χ^2 table on page 280. Like the t table, the column headings are .... and the rows correspond to different values of .... (symbol).

significance levels

f

20.11 Compare the structure of the χ^2 table with the t table. What is the important difference?

The χ^2 table presents values for significance levels of 0.99 and 0.95 as well as for 0.10, 0.05, 0.02 and 0.01.

20.12 The 0.99 and 0.95 levels correspond to the state of affairs where the observed results differ from the theoretical results *less* even than you would expect by chance. In 99 or 95 cases out of 100 such a result or a more extreme (i.e. more different from what is expected) result would occur by chance.
What does this imply for observed results that are even less different from the theoretical results?

The possibility of cheating. The result appears to be too good to be true!

20.13 In fact Mendel's pea observations based on genetic theory differed *less* than you would have expected by pure chance, $p > 0.95$. Do you think Mendel, an abbot, cheated?

He did not. In fact, it was subsequently found that the abbot's gardener knew the results the abbot wanted and tried to please him!

20.14 The main criteria for applying χ^2 are:
a) The samples are .... chosen.
b) The data are ....
c) Ideally the lowest expected frequency in any group is not less than 5. (This is now thought to be rather too conservative, and that even lower values can be allowed – for example, as low as 2, or even 1. But it is better to err on the conservative side, if at all.)

randomly
qualitative
N.B. Assume all the samples are random in this chapter.

20.15 One of the commonest reasons for using χ^2 is to see whether actual counts comply with those expected on theoretical grounds (*goodness of fit to a theory*). This is so with the example below based on genetic theory. Are all the criteria for applying χ^2 satisfied here?

Yes. The 3 criteria listed in the previous frame are satisfied. The lowest expected frequency is 25.

A geneticist was interested in seeing whether two plants had the genotype Aa. He crossed them to see how close the progeny were to the theoretical ratio:

$^1/_2$ Aa : $^1/_4$ AA : $^1/_4$ aa

There were 100 progeny (which may be considered to constitute a random sample of progeny from the two plants) and these were his results:

Genotype	Number observed (O)	Number expected on theory (E)
Aa	53	50
AA	23	25
aa	24	25
Total	100	100

20.16 In the last frame state the Null Hypothesis and its alternative.

Null Hypothesis: The differences are only due to chance.
Alternative Hypothesis: The differences are more than could be reasonably expected by chance alone.

20.17 We will use $\chi^2 =$

$\sum \dfrac{\text{(observed number } - \text{ expected number)}^2}{\text{expected number}}$,

which we may denote by $\sum \dfrac{(O - E)^2}{E}$

There is a value of $\dfrac{(O - E)^2}{E}$ for

each class. $\sum$ is ....
and means ....

capital sigma
add together

20.17 *cont'd*

Both positive and negative values of $(O - E)$ become positive when squared, so large differences in either direction contribute to large values of the χ^2 statistic. The appropriate test is therefore a one-tailed test. If a large probability (*p* value) is associated with a computed test statistic (say $p > 0.95$), this implies that the observed values are very close to the expected values (the value of the χ^2 test statistic is small), and this opens up the possibility that agreement is even better than could be expected by random variation alone – i.e. there is the suggestion that the observations may have been fixed in some way.

20.18 In Frame 20.15:

The calculated value of

$\chi^2 = \dfrac{(53 - 50)^2}{50}$ for genotype Aa

$+$? for genotype AA

$+$? for genotype aa

= which value?

$$+ \frac{(23 - 25)^2}{25} + \frac{(24 - 25)^2}{25}$$

$$= \frac{9}{50} + \frac{4}{25} + \frac{1}{25} = \frac{19}{50}$$

$$= 0.38$$

20.19 In Frame 20.15:
The calculated value of $\chi^2 = 0.38$.
To find the corresponding significant value (critical value) of χ^2 we need to know ....

f

20.20 Where χ^2 is used, as in Frame 20.15, to decide whether the actual results 'fit' some theory (in this case genetic) $f = k - 1$ where k is the number of classes.
In Frame 20.15

$f = $ ....

$3 - 1 = 2$ (There are 3 classes or genotypes.)

20.21 The research worker using χ^2 is nearly always interested in just one tail – the top one – i.e. he is interested in differences between observed and expected results and not in their

20.21 *cont'd*
agreement with one another (since, as we have seen, large differences in either direction contribute to large values of χ^2). This is/is not the case in Frame 20.15.

It is

20.22 The χ^2 table on page 280 records values of χ^2 for one-tailed significance levels, as it stands.

In Frame 20.15, $f = 2$
∴ Significant (critical) χ^2 = ...
(one tail)

$\chi^2 = 5.991$ at the 0.05 (5%) level
$\chi^2 = 9.210$ at the 0.01 (1%) level
(both one-tailed) from the table.

20.23 The calculated value of $\chi^2 = 0.38$ and is less than the significant (critical) value of χ^2 (at the 0.05 (5%) level). What is your conclusion?

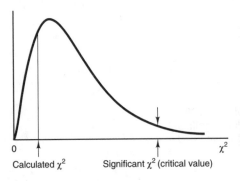

0 ↑   ↑
Calculated χ^2 Significant χ^2 (critical value)

Hint: The same as if the calculated value of *z* or *t* was less than the tabulated significant (critical) value of *z* or *t*.

You accept the Null Hypothesis. The conclusion is that the variation is insufficient to suspect that any other factor is involved and is due only to chance, i.e. the results 'fit' the genetic theory.

Note: Although this diagram indicates the general shape of the χ^2 distribution, for $f < 3$ the mode is in fact at the value zero, so here (with $f = 2$) the diagram is for illustrative purposes only.

Note also that the calculated value of χ^2 (0.38) is greater than 0.103, which is the tabulated value corresponding to a significance level of 0.95. There is therefore no reason to suspect fiddling of the results.

20.24 $f = n - 1$ in ordinary t tests where μ is known.

$f = k - 1$ in χ^2 testing 'goodness of fit' between actual results and results expected according to some theory. n in these t tests is the number of .... whereas in χ^2 k represents the number of ....

results

classes

20.25 $f = n - 1$ in the paired t-test also. Here n is the number of ....

differences

20.26 Suppose that the geneticist has performed another experiment. See below for details.
State the Null Hypothesis and the alternative.

Here he expected the two-factor segregation genetics ratio 9 AB : 3 Ab : 3 aB : 1 ab.
These are his results:

The Null Hypothesis is that the differences from what was expected are only due to chance. The alternative is that the variation is greater than that expected by chance alone.

Phenotype	Number observed (O)	Number expected (E)
AB	245	
Ab	80	
aB	70	
ab	5	
Total	400	

20.27 There are 400 offspring in the last frame. The expected numbers in each class are in the ratio 9 : 3 : 3 : 1.

So they are: AB?
Ab?
aB?
ab?

225	75	75	25
AB	Ab	aB	ab

i.e. 9 : 3 : 3 : 1

Use these expected values to obtain his conclusion in the next frame.

20.28 Can we apply χ^2 here?
The formula for χ^2 =

The calculated value of χ^2 = + + +
= ....?

Yes, because the lowest E = 25.

$$\Sigma \frac{(O - E)^2}{E}$$

20.28	*cont'd*	$= \dfrac{(254-225)^2}{225} + \dfrac{(80-75)^2}{75}$

$+ \dfrac{(70-75)^2}{75} + \dfrac{(5-25)^2}{25} = 18\dfrac{4}{9}$

$f = ?$
(one/two tails)?

$k - 1 = 3$
one tail

Significant (critical) $\chi^2 = ?$

7.815 for the 0.05 (5%) level
11.340 for the 0.01 (1%) level

So the conclusion is what?

$18\dfrac{4}{9}$ is very much larger than the significant (critical) value of χ^2. So we reject the Null Hypothesis. We conclude that there is more variation than you could reasonably expect by chance and that some further factor is involved (e.g. linking of genes) to produce the observed results.

When a difference like this is found the next stage would be to look back at the observed values and to see where the largest differences between those and the theoretical values occur. This can help to provide further useful information about the data.

20.29 So far the expected results were calculated on some theoretical grounds (genetic). Just as sometimes for calculating z we use .... to estimate σ^2, so sometimes for χ^2 we use the observed results (O) to estimate the expected results (E).

s^2
We use the observed results like this in testing whether one factor is *associated* with another.

20.30 When we use χ^2 to test *association* rather than to test *goodness of fit* to a theory it affects the value of f. What does f represent?

The number of degrees of freedom

20.31 The data to be tested for association are arranged in what is called a 'contingency table'. Here is an example. Is this a table of 'O's or 'E's?

In a survey to help decide whether a particular inoculation had any protective properties the following results were obtained for 300 people during an epidemic:

	Inoculated	Not inoculated	Row total
Affected	5	55	60
Not affected	95	145	240
Column total	100	200	300

Observed results ('O's)

This is the simplest form of contingency table. It is a two-way table (there are just two ways of classifying the people) with just two categories in each classification. Contingency tables can be more complex in two different ways:
1. There may be more ways of classifying the subjects (leading to three-way, four-way tables and so on). We will not deal with such tables here.
2. There may be more than two categories in one or more of the classifications.

20.32 State the Null Hypothesis and its alternative here.

The Null Hypothesis is that any association is due to chance only.
The alternative is that an association really exists between inoculation and incidence. (If so, we would expect inoculation to protect people against the disease.) Inspection of the data will then reveal the direction of the association.

20.33 We assume initially that the Null Hypothesis/Alternative Hypothesis is true and on this basis calculate the expected results using the row and column totals.

Null Hypothesis

20.34 In Frame 20.31, using the column totals, we see that 100 out of the total 300, or 1/3, were inoculated. Assuming the Null Hypothesis is true and that inoculation is not really associated with the incidence of the disease, we would expect 1/3 of those affected to have been inoculated/not inoculated.

Inoculated, i.e. 1/3 of the people are inoculated and as this is assumed to have had no effect, 1/3 of those affected would be inoculated.

20.35 But in Frame 20.31 we see that a total of 60 people are affected. Therefore we would expect that .... of them had been inoculated.

1/3, or 20

20.36 Similarly 2/3 of the total are not inoculated and so you would expect 2/3 of those 60 affected, i.e. 40 people to be affected and inoculated/not inoculated.

not inoculated

20.37 As inoculation is assumed to have no effect and 1/3 are inoculated, you would expect also 1/3 of the 240 not affected to be inoculated.
That is, you would expect .... inoculated, not affected people.

$1/3 \times 240 = 80$

20.38 The expected results calculated in the last 3 frames are shown below. How many not inoculated, not affected people would you expect?

2/3 of those not affected i.e. 2/3 of 240 = 160

	Inoculated	Not inoculated
Affected	20	40
Not affected	80	?

20.39 The contingency tables for the observed results and for the expected results are shown below:

Observed (O):

	Inoculated	Not inoculated	Row total
Affected	5	55	60
Not affected	95	145	240
Column total	100	200	300

20.39 *cont'd*
Expected (*E*):

	Inoculated	Not inoculated	Row total
Affected	20	40	60
Not affected	80	160	240
Column total	100	200	300

What do you notice about the row totals and column totals in each table?

They are the same in both tables.

20.40 Also notice that each expected result equals

its row total × its column total

the overall total

For example, for the inoculated, affected group in Frame 20.39 the expected result

$$= \frac{? \times 100}{?} = 20$$

$$\frac{60 \times 100}{300} = 20$$

20.41 How can you calculate the expected frequencies in contingency tables?

Use the formula:

$$\frac{\text{row total} \times \text{column total}}{\text{grand total}}$$

20.42 Give the three criteria for applying a χ^2 test. They are: The data are .... and the samples are .... and no expected frequency is less than ....

qualitative
random
5 (though, remember, this is quite conservative).

20.43 Can χ^2 be applied to our inoculation data here?

'*O*':

	Inoculated	Not inoculated	Row total
Affected	5	55	60
Not affected	95	145	240
Column total	100	200	300

Yes, provided that the samples are random, since no expected result is less than 5.

20.43   *cont'd*
      'E':

	Inoculated	Not inoculated	Row total
Affected	20	40	60
Not affected	80	160	240
Column total	100	200	300

20.44   Remember we were interested to see whether the inoculation protected against the disease. We expect, if this is so, to observe fewer inoculated, affected people than expected. Are there? Otherwise we must reject the theory immediately.

Yes
20 were expected but only 5 were observed in this group. We can now go on to use the χ^2 test to see whether the *differences* are greater than could be expected by random variation alone.

  Is the χ^2 test a one- or a two-tailed test?

A one-tailed test (as is usual for a contingency table test)

20.45   What is the formula for calculating χ^2?

$$\chi^2 = \sum \frac{(O - E)^2}{E}$$

20.46   In Frame 20.43
$$\chi^2 = \frac{(5 - 20)^2}{20} + ? + ? + ?$$
$$= ?$$

$$+ \frac{(55 - 40)^2}{40} + \frac{(95 - 80)^2}{80}$$
$$+ \frac{(145 - 160)^2}{160}$$
$$= \frac{3375}{160} \approx 21$$

20.47   When χ^2 was used to test 'goodness of fit' to a theory $f =$

$k - 1$

20.48   In using χ^2 to test association in a contingency table $f = (r - 1)(c - 1)$, where r is the number of rows and c is the number of columns in the body of the table.

  Hence, in Frame 20.43, $f = ?$

$(2 - 1)(2 - 1) = 1$

20.49   That is, there is one degree of freedom.

This is because if one expected result is calculated in a 2-rowed, 2-columned contingency table (what is called a 2×2 table), as the row and column totals are fixed, the rest of the numbers in the table cannot be chosen freely.

As an example complete this fictitious table:

	B	Not B	Row total
A	10	?	40
Not A	?	?	85
Column total	50	75	125

	B	Not B	Row total
A	10	40−10 = 30	40
Not A	50−10 = 40	75−30 = 45	85
Column total	50	75	125

This is an example where there is only one free choice (one degree of freedom).

20.50   Anyway, to come back to the inoculation problem:
In Frame 20.44 you decided this was a .... tailed test.
In Frame 20.48 you calculated f to equal ....
Hence, what are the required significant (critical) χ^2 values in the table?

one

one
3.841 for the 0.05 (5%) level
6.635 for the 0.01 (1%) level

20.51   In Frame 20.46 χ^2 was calculated from the contingency tables to be equal to 21. What is your conclusion, therefore?

The Null Hypothesis is rejected. We saw that fewer people who were inoculated got the disease (confirmed by inspection of the data). Now we can add that the degree of protection is statistically significant ($p < 0.01$).

20.52   When χ^2 is used to test 'goodness of fit' to a theory (e.g. genetics), $f = ?$

$k - 1$, where k is the number of classes

20.53 For testing for *goodness of fit* to a theory, the theory itself is used to calculate the expected results. However, to use χ^2 to test for *association* we use the observed results to calculate the expected values and $f = ?$

$(r - 1)(c - 1)$, where r is the number of rows and c is the number of columns in the contingency table.

20.54 In testing for association we calculated the expected values using which formula?

$$\frac{\text{row total} \times \text{column total}}{\text{grand total}}$$

20.55 Calculate the expected contingency table for these observed results:

'O'		Hair colour Fair	Dark	
Eye	Blue	23	12	35
colour	Green	2	3	5
	Brown	15	45	60
		40	60	100

'E'		Fair	Dark	
Eye	Blue			
colour	Green			
	Brown			

Using

$$E = \frac{\text{row total} \times \text{column total}}{\text{grand total}},$$

the table of expected frequencies is as follows:

14	21	35
2	3	5
24	36	60
40	60	100

What is the value of f for this contingency table? Can χ^2 be applied here?

$f = (3 - 1)(2 - 1) = 2$
Strictly speaking, no, since there are too few green-eyed people. But, given that the requirement that the smallest expected value is 5 is somewhat conservative, this table is about at the limit of acceptability for using χ^2.

20.56 We can adjust this by pooling the blue- and green-eyed people, for example. (We might alternatively have pooled the green- and brown-eyed people.) Thus:

'O'		Hair colour Fair	Dark	
Eye	Blue or			
colour	green	25	15	40
	Brown	15	45	60
		40	60	100

20.56 *cont'd*
What is the expected contingency table now?

'E'		Hair colour Fair	Dark
Eye colour	Blue or green		
	Brown		

16	24	40
24	36	60
40	60	100

What is *f* now?
Can χ^2 be applied here now?

$f = (2 - 1)(2 - 1) = 1$
Yes, the lowest *E* is now 16. (Pooling results sometimes enables χ^2 to be applicable. The groups which are pooled are small and they are combined with others similar to themselves.) Note, however, that the choice of pooling may not be unique. (Pooling should, however, always be carried out, if at all, in a meaningful way.) For example, we could have pooled green-eyed and brown-eyed people in the above table. This can lead to numerically different results – even though the broad conclusions may be (but need not necessarily be) the same, whichever choice of pooling is adopted.

20.57 $\chi^2 = \sum \dfrac{(O - E)^2}{E}$
= ? in the last frame?

$\dfrac{(25 - 16)^2}{16} + \dfrac{(15 - 24)^2}{24}$

$+ \dfrac{(15 - 24)^2}{24} + \dfrac{(45 - 36)^2}{36}$

$\simeq 14$

20.58 Assuming this is a one-tailed test with $f = 1$, then the significant value (critical value) of χ^2 from the χ^2 tables is?

3.841 for the 0.05 (5%) level
6.635 for the 0.01 (1%) level

20.59 What is your conclusion?

The calculated value of χ^2 is bigger than the tabulated values at both the 5% and 1% levels. Hence, the Null Hypothesis is rejected. There is a significant association between eye colour and hair colour ($p < 0.01$). Inspection of the data will now reveal the nature of that association.

20.60 What is the value of f in a 3-row × 8-column contingency table (referred to as a 3 × 8 table) for testing for association?

$(3 - 1)(8 - 1) = 14$

20.61 By completing the answers below decide whether you think that knowledge of bilharzia protects children from risking contracting the disease.
Here are the results obtained by Dr Bill:

The Null Hypothesis is that any association is due to chance only.
The alternative is that there is an association between knowledge and risk and inspection of the data would then reveal the nature of the association.

	No knowledge	Some knowledge	Good knowledge	Row total
No risk	20	40	20	80
Definite risk	40	60	20	120
Column total	60	100	40	200

State the Null Hypothesis and the alternative, calculating the expected table using the formula:
$E =$

We find:

$$E = \frac{\text{row total} \times \text{column total}}{\text{grand total}}$$

	No knowledge	Some knowledge	Good knowledge	Row total
No risk	24	40	16	80
Definite risk	36	60	24	120
Column total	60	100	40	200

20.61 *cont'd*
We can/cannot use χ^2

$\chi^2 =$ which formula?
$\chi^2 =$ which value?

$$\chi^2 = \sum \frac{(O - E)^2}{E}$$

$$= \frac{(20 - 24)^2}{24} + \frac{(40 - 40)^2}{40}$$

$$+ \frac{(20 - 16)^2}{16}$$

$$+ \frac{(40 - 36)^2}{36} + \frac{(60 - 60)^2}{60}$$

$$+ \frac{(20 - 24)^2}{24}$$

$$= 2\frac{7}{9}$$

$$(2 - 1)(3 - 1) = 2$$

$f = ?$

This is a one-/two-tailed test?

One. Notice those who have good knowledge take less risks than expected. But is this difference large enough to be due to anything more than chance variation?

The significant (critical) value of $\chi^2 = ?$

5.991 for the 0.05 (5%) level
9.210 for the 0.01 (1%) level

The conclusion is what?

Either knowledge does not protect or there is insufficient evidence to show that it does.

What should Dr Bill do?
He was thinking of employing a Health Educator.

Increase the numbers observed to distinguish between these two possibilities, or do not employ such a person.

20.62 If Dr Bill had calculated χ^2 as 0.019 ($f = 2$), what idea should have entered your head?

This value is less than the 0.99 and 0.95 significant (critical) values. You should have suspected cheating – it is difficult to believe that a result so close to that expected could have occurred in practice.

20.63 What is the formula used for f if testing for association?

$f = (r - 1)(c - 1)$

20.64 What is the value of f if χ^2 is used for testing 'goodness of fit' to a theory?

$f = k - 1$

20.65 What are the criteria for employing a χ^2 test?

The samples are random. The data are qualitative. No E is less than 5 (conservative rule).

20.66 If some values of E are much less than 5 and the contingency table is large, how can you sometimes overcome this obstacle?

By pooling some classes as we did in Frame 20.56. If there is 1 degree of freedom, particularly if some of the E values are small, we should, in theory, apply a correction (called Yates's correction) – but we will not deal with this any further here.

20.67 Otherwise what is the formula for χ^2?

$$\chi^2 = \Sigma \frac{(O - E)^2}{E}$$

20.68 **Practical example**
Mr Place wants to know whether malignancy is associated with the site of cerebral tumours.
His results were:

See page 260.

	Benign	Malignant	
Frontal lobe	21	19	40
Temporal lobe	28	2	30
Other lobes	51	29	80
	100	50	150

What conclusion would he draw?

SUMMARY

χ^2 (chi-squared) is the distribution used for hypotheses about data where:
1. The samples are random.
2. The data are qualitative.
3. There is ideally no expected value less than 5.

The calculated value of $\chi^2 = \sum \dfrac{(O - E)^2}{E}$, where O and E denote observed and expected results respectively.

For one-tailed tests (which are usual when carrying out χ^2 tests) values of χ^2 given in the table in this book are used directly. As always in such situations, if you are using tables from some other source, look carefully to see exactly what is being tabulated. If it is found that the calculated value of χ^2 is less than the tabulated 0.95 or 0.99 values it suggests the possibility of cheating. $f = k - 1$ where k is the number of classes if testing 'goodness of fit to a theory'.

Where χ^2 is used to test for associations in a contingency table, the expected results are calculated using

$$E = \frac{\text{row total} \times \text{column total}}{\text{grand total}}$$

Here $f = (r - 1)(c - 1)$, where r is the number of rows and c is the number of columns in the body of the contingency table.

The Null Hypothesis states that the differences between the observed and expected results are due to chance variation only. If the calculated value of χ^2 is greater than the significant (critical) value of χ^2, the Null Hypothesis is rejected.

21. **Nonparametric methods**

INTRODUCTION

So far we have dealt with methods of statistical analysis which are based in some way on an assumed model for the data (e.g. the data have a normal distribution), which, in turn, is specified in terms of one or more parameters (e.g. mean μ and variance σ^2 of the normal distribution). However, we saw in Chapter 19, in the context of simple linear regression, that it is not always reasonable to make such an assumption. One possibility then is to have recourse to a transformation of the data, in the hope that the transformed data will satisfy the assumptions. An alternative is to have recourse to nonparametric methods, which are based on far weaker assumptions. They are sometimes called distribution-free methods, for a self-explanatory reason.

21.1	We have met a number of statistical tests so far. What have the tests been based upon?	A model for the data (e.g. the underlying data are normally distributed)
21.2	The underlying model assumed for an observed set of data in a statistical test is specified by what?	By its parameters (e.g. the mean μ and variance σ^2 of the normal distribution)
21.3	What do you then need to state, in order to be able to carry out the test?	A Null Hypothesis and an Alternative Hypothesis. These are stated in terms of a parameter of the model. For example we might have: Null Hypothesis: $\mu = 0$ Alternative Hypothesis: $\mu \neq 0$ (e.g. for matched pairs, when testing for a non-zero mean difference)
21.4	If the assumptions of the model are not satisfied by the data, what might you do to rectify this situation?	Transform the data
21.5	If you want to render non-normally distributed data normally distributed, what is often a useful transformation to try?	A logarithmic transformation

21.6	Rather than carry out a transformation of the data, what might you otherwise try?	A nonparametric method

21.7   In Chapter 15 we were introduced to the ideas of significance testing through the example concerning males and females contracting a particular complication of bilharzia. The ideas involved there are similar to the ideas that we need again now. Consider the following, similar example.

21.8   Suppose that two treatments, A and B, for some medical condition are being compared in a small study involving 8 subjects. Each subject received both treatments. A very simple assessment is made, in which each subject is required to express a preference for one treatment or the other. Assume that strict preferences only are allowed (i.e. 'A is better than B' or 'B is better than A'); a verdict of 'no preference' is not allowed (although this would often be a legitimate third category).

What is the appropriate Null Hypothesis for the test that needs to be carried out?

Null Hypothesis: Probability that A is preferred to B = Probability that B is preferred to A = $1/2$.

21.9   What would an appropriate Alternative Hypothesis be?

There is no indication that any preference is only anticipated in one direction, so a two-sided alternative is appropriate. We have: Alternative Hypothesis: Probability that A is preferred to B $\neq$ Probability that B is preferred to A.

21.10   Suppose that 6 subjects express a preference for treatment A, while 2 subjects express a preference for treatment B. What is the probability of this outcome, if the Null Hypothesis is true?

The probability of this outcome is

$$\binom{8}{6} \left(\frac{1}{2}\right)^6 \left(\frac{1}{2}\right)^8$$

21.10   *cont'd*

$$= \frac{(8 \times 7)}{(1 \times 2)} \left(\frac{1}{2}\right)^8$$

$$= \frac{28}{2^8} = \frac{7}{64} = 0.1094$$

This result requires some explanation! Denoting preference for treatment A by A and for treatment B by B, one sequence of interest is A A A A A A B B. By the multiplication law of probability, this event has probability

$$\left(\frac{1}{2}\right)^6 \left(\frac{1}{2}\right)^2 = \left(\frac{1}{2}\right)^8.$$

But the order of the A's and B's does not matter, just so long as there are 6 A's and 2 B's. It is the number of ways of doing this that is denoted by

$\binom{8}{6}$. Think of putting

the 2 B's into 2 of the 8 positions in the sequence of 8. This is the simpler way to approach it, and leads us towards the number of ways of choosing 2 objects out of

8, denoted by $\binom{8}{2}$,

which can then be seen to be exactly the same as

$\binom{8}{6}$. The first B can be

put in any one of 8 positions, and the second B can be put in any one of the remaining 7 positions,

making $8 \times 7 = 56$

21.10 *cont'd*

possibilities altogether. But this doubles up on the number of different arrangements of A's and B's of interest. This is because there is no difference between putting the first B in position 8 and the second B in position 7, for example, and putting the first B in position 7 and the second B in position 8.

Another way of looking at this which helps in the more general case where there are more than 2 B's is to note that one of the two remaining positions for the first B can be chosen in 2 ways, leaving just 1 way to choose the position for the second B: i.e. 2×1 ways altogether. So the number of different arrangements of this type

reduces to $\dfrac{(8 \times 7)}{(1 \times 2)} = 28$.

This is often represented,

as above, by $\begin{pmatrix} 8 \\ 2 \end{pmatrix}$, the

number of ways of choosing 2 positions in the sequence from 8, and is called a *binomial coefficient*. As we have seen, this is the same

as $\begin{pmatrix} 8 \\ 6 \end{pmatrix}$. For those of you

who go on to read about specific probability distributions, this is central to the binomial distribution.

21.11 Is this the probability that you need in order to be able to decide on the result of the hypothesis test?

No, on its own it is not. Something more is required.

21.12 In words, what is the probability that is required for carrying out the hypothesis test?

It is the probability of the result observed, or of one more extreme. Since we are concerned with a two-sided alternative this means more extreme in either direction.

21.13 What is the required probability numerically?

It is

$$2\left[\binom{8}{6}\left(\frac{1}{2}\right)^6\left(\frac{1}{2}\right)^2\right.$$
$$+\binom{8}{7}\left(\frac{1}{2}\right)^7\left(\frac{1}{2}\right)$$
$$\left.+\binom{8}{8}\left(\frac{1}{2}\right)^8\right].$$

The term inside the square brackets is the probability of 6 preferences for A and 2 for B, or 7 preferences for A and 1 for B, or all 8 preferences for A (formed by adding together the probabilities of mutually exclusive events). This probability is then multiplied by 2 to take account of the equally extreme result in the opposite direction, with the same probability numerically, namely of 6 preferences for B and 2 for A, or 7 preferences for B and 1 for A, or all 8 preferences for B. The above probability reduces to:

$$\frac{2}{2^8}\left[\frac{8\times7}{1\times2}+8+1\right]$$

$$=\frac{37}{2^7}=\frac{37}{128}=0.2891.$$

21.14 So what is the outcome of the hypothesis test?

Working at the 0.05, or 5%, level of significance the result is not significant ($p = 0.2891$, so $p > 0.05$).

21.14	*cont'd*	Either there is no difference between the treatments or there is insufficient evidence to show the difference.
21.15	How else might you have quoted the outcome of the test?	The *p* value associated with the observed outcome is 0.29.
21.16	What is preferable about this second way of expressing the outcome?	It is more informative. It does not just tell us that the result is significant or not significant at a particular level, but also how close to that level it is.
21.17	So far this is really just revision of what we have done before (in Chapter 15). However, that in itself serves to emphasise that the principles involved here are just the same as they were there. Before we leave this introductory example let us consider an amendment to it. Suppose in a similar treatment comparison there are only 5 subjects involved and that all 5 express a preference for A. What is the probability of this extreme event, or the extreme one in the other direction?	It is $$2\left(\frac{1}{2}\right)^5 = \frac{1}{16} = 0.0625.$$
21.18	So, working with a two-tailed test, is this result significant at the 5% level?	No, it is not.
21.19	With just 5 subjects in the study, what outcome, in a two-tailed test, would be significant at the 5% level?	None would. We have observed the most extreme result possible, in terms of preference for one treatment over the other. There is nothing more extreme which would reduce the *p* value. (Of course, if a one-tailed test had been appropriate, it would be a different matter.)

21.20 What lesson is there to be learnt from this?

Small samples yield low power to detect differences, even when they exist. In this last example, the difference can never be detected at the 5% significance level, even with the most extreme outcome possible.

21.21 An alternative way of labelling the outcomes in the simple example we have been studying would have been to designate 'A preferred to B' by $+$ and 'B preferred to A' by $-$. The outcome from the group of size 8 could then be depicted as $+ + + + +\.+ - -$. Not surprisingly, the name given to the type of test we have just been using is the *sign test*. It is the simplest type of nonparametric test.

21.22 In a (fictitious) study concerning a treatment for chronic pain, 12 patients recorded their level of pain on a 10 cm long visual analogue scale. They did this upon entry to the study, and again after one week's treatment. The following differences in cm between second and first pain measures for each patient were recorded (negative differences imply an improvement in pain level):
-1.2, -2.3, $+2.6$, -4.1, -0.7, -2.1, $+1.8$, $+0.9$, -1.3, -3.5, -2.0, -1.9.
If you were going to carry out a sign test on these data, how could you represent the data?

The data could be represented as follows:
$- - + - - - + + - -$
$- -$

21.23 Why might you not wish to do this?

Representing the data in this way, and carrying out a test simply on the signs, constitutes a quite drastic reduction of the data and a discarding of information. We should not do this lightly. Even if we are not prepared to make distributional assumptions

21.23	*cont'd*	about the data, we should try to utilise the information concerning the magnitude of the differences.
21.24	Do you know another name for nonparametric methods?	Probably not yet. They are also called distribution-free methods.
21.25	How does this name come about?	No distributional assumption is made about the underlying data.
21.26	We are about to meet the Wilcoxon matched-pairs signed-ranks test. In what context have we already met ranked data?	In the computation of Spearman's rank correlation coefficient.
21.27	The Wilcoxon matched-pairs signed-ranks test is not completely distribution-free. It depends for its validity on the assumption that the underlying distribution of the data is *symmetric*. Note that this is not such a strong assumption as that the data are normally distributed (which would be the corresponding assumption for a parametric, or classical, method). Is the assumption satisfied for our data?	With only 12 values it is difficult to decide whether or not it is reasonable to assume a symmetric distribution. However, a check of the data does not reveal any problem in this respect. (Note that with so few data values, it is difficult to do anything else as a check other than to inspect the data.)
21.28	Parametric, or classical, tests relating to the centre of a distribution are concerned with the mean. Can you suggest what measure of central tendency nonparametric tests are concerned with?	The median
21.29	In the example we are considering, concerning a treatment for chronic pain, what would be a suitable Null Hypothesis for the test?	A suitable Null Hypothesis would be that there is no difference in pain level, before and after treatment. More precisely, this can be stated as the median difference is zero.

21.30 Again, in the example we are considering, is a one-sided or two-sided Alternative Hypothesis appropriate?

A one-sided Alternative Hypothesis is appropriate. In a study of *chronic* pain we cannot contemplate how an active treatment could make the pain level worse. (Though note that often in medical work a two-sided Alternative Hypothesis is used, even when a one-sided alternative might seem to be indicated. This provides a more conservative approach. This is a remark about tests generally, not just nonparametric tests.)

21.31 State an appropriate Alternative Hypothesis.

The pain level after treatment is lower than that before treatment. More precisely, the median difference in pain level, comparing pain after treatment with that before, is less than zero.

21.32 Given the Alternative Hypothesis that you have stated would you anticipate fewer negative or positive differences in the data?

Fewer positive differences are anticipated, because these correspond to increase in pain level.

21.33 As the name of the test suggests, the Wilcoxon matched-pairs signed-ranks test is based on ranks. Rank the observed differences from 1 to 12, in order of magnitude, starting with the smallest, and ignoring the signs of the differences.

We have the following:

Difference	Rank
−1.2	3
−2.3	9
+2.6	10
−4.1	12
−0.7	1
−2.1	8
+1.8	5
+0.9	2
−1.3	4
−3.5	11
−2.0	7
−1.9	6

21.34 Suppose that two of the differences had been numerically the same (but possibly with different signs attached), e.g. +1.9, −1.9 (rather than +1.8, −1.9). Then these values would each be assigned the average of the ranks that they would otherwise have received. What, therefore, would the ranks be?

These two values would have occupied the ranks 5 and 6. The average of these is 5.5, so this is the rank that would be assigned to each of +1.9, −1.9.

21.35 If any of the differences are zero, ignore those data and reduce the sample size accordingly.

21.36 We now need to construct the test statistic. The Wilcoxon signed-rank statistic T is the sum of the ranks of *either* the positive differences *or* the negative differences, *whichever the one-sided Alternative Hypothesis suggests should be the smaller*. Calculate the test statistic T in the present example.

The Alternative Hypothesis indicates that the sum of the positive differences should be the smaller. We therefore need to add together the ranks associated with the following differences:
+2.6, +1.8, +0.9
Hence,
$T = 10 + 5 + 2 = 17$

21.37 Explain in words the principle of what needs to be done with this test statistic to arrive at a conclusion for the hypothesis test.

The computed value of the test statistic needs to be compared with the reference distribution. We no longer have a standard theoretical distribution (e.g. the normal distribution) underlying the test statistic. Rather, we have all the possible values of T arising from permuting + and − signs in all possible ways amongst the ranks. For this reason the distribution is called a *permutation distribution*.

There is interest, then, in the usual way, in the probability of a result as extreme or more extreme than the observed one.

21.38 You may be somewhat daunted by the thought of needing to compute a permutation distribution each time you want to carry out a test like this.	Do not worry! It has all been done for you, and the results of the calculations appear in tables of the T statistic.
21.39 If the computed value of T is less than or equal to the tabulated value then the result is significant at the chosen level. Carry out the test for the present example, using the 5% significance level.	From the table of the T statistic, for $n = 12$, $\alpha_1 = 5\%$ (giving a one-tailed test value) the significant (critical) value is 17. The calculated value of T from the data is also 17, so the result is just significant at the 5% level. The treatment is effective at reducing the pain level.
21.40 On another occasion we may have been interested in carrying out a two-sided test. The procedure then is to define as the test statistic T the smaller of the two computed rank sums. The value in the table to compare this with is then the one corresponding to α_2. So if this had been the case in the example we were considering ($n = 12$), the significant (critical) value would have been 13 (see the table) and the result would not have been significant at the 5% level.	
21.41 What parametric test do you think the Wilcoxon matched-pairs signed-ranks T test corresponds to?	The matched-pairs t-test.
21.42 You may ask why we do not *always* use a nonparametric method, if we do not have to worry about strong distributional assumptions for the data.	The answer is that if we apply a nonparametric test in a situation where the corresponding parametric (classical) test is valid, the nonparametric test will be less efficient than the parametric (classical) test. Some of the nonparametric methods do compare very favourably, however, even when the parametric (classical) methods are valid.

21.43 We have been looking at the nonparametric equivalent to the matched-pairs t-test. Another type of t-test that we have met is the two-sample test for comparing means of samples. We will now look at the nonparametric equivalent to that, but for comparing the medians of two samples rather than the means. The test is called the Mann–Whitney U-test.

21.44 Consider here another example involving pain scores, as recorded on a 10 cm visual analogue scale. Suppose that a new analgesic is being compared with placebo in the treatment of post-operative pain following some surgical procedure. Eleven patients entered the study and were allocated randomly to receive active treatment or placebo. The pain scores recorded by the patients 4 hours after the operation were as follows:

Active: 2.4 3.2 1.2 2.3 1.4
Placebo: 3.6 2.8 4.1 3.4 3.1 3.9

21.45 What is an appropriate Null Hypothesis to be tested?

There is no difference between the median pain levels in the two treatment groups.

21.46 What is an appropriate Alternative Hypothesis against which to test?

The median pain level for the active treatment group is lower than the median pain level for the placebo group.

21.47 Is the test, as defined by the responses to Frames 21.44 and 21.45, one-sided or two-sided?

It is one-sided. We do not anticipate that patients could experience more pain because of receiving active treatment, compared with receiving an inactive treatment (placebo).

21.48   Describe in words the principles underlying the test we should carry out.

As usual we will compute an appropriate test statistic for showing up the type of difference we are interested in, then we will compare it with the known distribution of the test statistic under the Null Hypothesis. We will then consider the probability associated with an outcome as extreme as or more extreme than the one observed.

21.49   Denoting the active treatment group by A and the placebo group by P, arrange all the data in ascending order, labelling each data point with an A or P.

1.2 1.4 2.3 2.4 2.8 3.1
 A   A   A   A   P   P
3.2 3.4 3.6 3.9 4.1
 A   P   P   P   P

21.50   Now write out just the letter sequence obtained from Frame 21.49.

A A A A P P
A P P P P

21.51   Now write under each A the number of Ps that precede it in the sequence.

A A A A P P
0 0 0 0
A P P P P
2

21.52   Under the Null Hypothesis we expect the number of times an A value is preceded by a P value to be small. This is indeed the way it has turned out, so what remains to be done?

We need to decide *how small* is the number of times an A value is preceded by a P value, compared with what we could expect by random variation alone, if there really is not any difference between the median of the A and P values; i.e. is the number significantly small?

21.53   The Mann–Whitney U-statistic is now simply the sum of the separate numbers of times that an A value is preceded by a P value. Compute the U-statistic.

The U-statistic for this example is given by:
$0 + 0 + 0 + 0 + 2 = 2$

21.54 If there are any tied observations in the different groups, assign 1/2 to the count of the total number of times an A value is preceded by a P value, for each tied pair. What is the score for the number of times an A is preceded by a P in the following sequence, where the boxed values are tied?

A A | A A P | A P | A P | P

The score is
$U = 0 + 0 + {}^1/_2 + {}^1/_2 + 1 + 2{}^1/_2 = 4{}^1/_2$

21.55 Returning to the data in Frames 21.44 and 21.49, compute a corresponding statistic U^*, where U^* is the sum of the separate numbers of times that a P value is preceded by an A value.

This time we have

A	A	A	A	P
				4
P	A	P	P	P
4		5	5	5
P				
5				

So $U^* = 4 + 4 + 5 + 5 + 5 + 5 = 28$

21.56 The test statistic we need (out of U and U^*) is the one corresponding to the smaller count as anticipated under the Null Hypothesis.

Note that we should usually be able to see from the data which way round we need to be looking at the data to compute the test statistic, as above. The position may not always be so clear-cut, though.

21.57 Frames 21.53 and 21.55 show that even if we cannot spot which of U and U^* is going to be the smaller, we could compute the two values, then use the smaller one (as long as it is in the direction of the Alternative Hypothesis – in this case, smaller median corresponding to A). But even this is not necessary.

21.58 The two values U, U^* are connected by the relationship $U = n_A n_P - U^*$ where n_A, n_P are the sizes of the active treatment and placebo groups, respectively. In Frame 21.53 we computed U as 2. What are n_A and n_P, and so what is U^*?

$n_A = 5$
$n_P = 6$
$U^* = (5 \times 6) - 2 = 30 - 2 = 28$
This agrees with the computation in Frame 21.55.

21.59 As usual, the distribution of U has already been worked out for us, and the key features of it are tabulated. The complete distribution in our example with 5 A values and 6 P values comes about from permuting the positions of the A's and P's amongst the 11 ordered positions in the sequence.

What type of distribution is this?

A permutation distribution

21.60 In the tables we are concerned for significance with values of the observed test statistic U which are less than or equal to the tabulated significant value (critical value) at the chosen significance level. Noting that n_1 is the smaller of n_A and n_P, and n_2 is the other group size, we find that the critical value at the 5% significance level for a one-sided test (corresponding to α_1), for $n_1 = 5$ and $n_2 = 6$, is 5. At the 1% significance level it is 2. What is your conclusion?

The observed result is certainly significant at the 5% level, and also just at the 1% level.

21.61 In the above example we were only concerned with the outcome that the active treatment was more effective than the placebo as an alternative to the hypothesis that they were equally effective – and hence a one-sided test. In other situations we might be interested in what kind of test instead?

A two-sided test

21.62 In order to carry out a two-sided Mann–Whitney U-test the procedure is as follows. Compute the two values U and U^*. Do this by counting the total number of times A values precede B values, or the total number of times B values precede A values (denoting the two groups by A and B now), then by computing the other value from the relationship $U = n_A\, n_B - U^*$.
The *smaller* of the two values U and U^* is then used as the test statistic, and compared with the tabulated values, now using α_2 values.

21.63 Suppose that, rather than a placebo, the treatment other than A in the example in Frame 21.44 was another active treatment. Using the same results as in Frame 21.44 carry out a two-sided test of the hypothesis that the two treatments are equally effective.

We have already seen that the two values U and U^* are 2 and 28. Clearly the smaller value of the two is 2. Comparing with the tabulated critical values (3 at the 5% level, 1 at the 1% level), we find that the result is still significant at the 5% level, but not any more at the 1% level.

21.64 There is a Wilcoxon version of this Mann–Whitney test, which you may see referred to in textbooks. The statistics corresponding to U and U^* are then expressed in the form $R_A - \frac{1}{2}n_A (n_A + 1)$ and $R_B - \frac{1}{2}n_B (n_B + 1)$. We will not, however, look at that version of the test any further here, except to note that R_A and R_B are the sum of the ranks of the A's and the sum of the ranks of the B's, respectively, when all the A's and B's are listed in an ordered sequence, and n_A and n_B are the numbers of A's and B's respectively.

SUMMARY

Nonparametric methods, which are based on weak distributional assumptions about the underlying data (e.g. the distribution is symmetrical) or no distributional assumption at all, provide an alternative approach to significance testing when standard assumptions for a set of data (e.g. normal distribution) break down.

Two particularly useful nonparametric tests are the Wilcoxon matched-pairs signed-ranks test and the Mann–Whitney U-test. These are the nonparametric equivalents of the matched-pairs t-test and the two-sample t-test for comparing means, respectively, amongst the standard parametric tests (or z tests if the variances are known).

The nonparametric test statistics are based on the ordered data, and tabulated critical values of the test statistics are derived from permutation distributions.

22. Some brief remarks on statistical computing

Any of the computations covered in this programmed learning text can be easily carried out using a calculator. Actually, working with the data in this way leads to a good feel for the data and a thorough understanding of the principles involved in the computations. Some of you may never need to approach statistics in any different way from this, especially if the key requirement for you is an understanding of what statistics is all about, rather than carrying out computations yourselves. However, statistical computer packages are very widely used nowadays and many of you undoubtedly will go on to use these tools when you come to carry out your own analyses.

What is around to be used? In the pharmaceutical industry and in support to that industry, much of the statistical work is done within the SAS statistical computer package. This runs on mainframe machines and there is a personal computer version of it also. It is, however, somewhat expensive, which precludes its use amongst individuals and small groups. Other large and well-established packages are BMDP and SPSS. A package such as Minitab is suitable for carrying out a wide range of standard statistical analyses and has the benefits of being relatively cheap and self-teaching, with plenty of on-line help within the package. Indeed, for all-purpose statistical analyses, for wide-ranging applications (including medical), there are very many statistical computer packages around, which can be run on personal computers. Some other packages tend to be for particular, specialised types of analysis (for example, Egret for survival analysis).

Statistical computer packages need to be used with great caution, especially by those who do not have a proper understanding of the statistical analyses that they are trying to carry out with the packages. Computer packages always *appear* to produce very convincing output. It is all nicely printed out and *looks* correct. But if an analysis has been wrongly applied, or is an inappropriate analysis for the data, the results might actually be worthless. In many ways, statistical packages nowadays are *too* easy to use, since they contain many pitfalls for the unwary. A project undertaken some years ago at the University of Kent serves to illustrate this point. A regression package, U-REG, was developed there on behalf of a company which wanted to use the software for its scientists, who were carrying out lots of regression analyses, but who were not talking to the company statisticians about them. Now this may not sound very remarkable. Regression analysis is a very commonly used statistical technique and facilities for it exist in most standard statistical computer packages. But despite being so readily available, the technique is fraught with potential problems for those who are not thoroughly familiar with what they are doing. All sorts of problems can arise with the data, which may remain undetected by an inexpert user. What makes U-REG different from other regression packages or modules is that it detects any problems with the data, or other noteworthy features of them, and informs the user about them, through on-line dialogue. Without this type of safeguard the scientists may have been making a nonsense of the data through their attempts at proper analyses. So the advice is clear. Use statistical computer packages with care. Approach the analyses you are undertaking with thought, having due regard for any assumptions that need to be met by the data to render the analysis valid. Consult with a statistician if you need to, for example if you are unsure whether what you are doing is correct.

Much of what we have covered in this programmed learning text has concerned hypothesis testing and comparison of test statistics computed from the data with tabulated values from the theoretical distribution of the test statistic. Typically, the comparison is at a number of standard significance levels – e.g. 5%, 1%, 0.1%. But the computer can hold very detailed information from the full distribution. It is therefore an easy matter to produce a p value corresponding to a set of data under a particular Null Hypothesis. This is, as we have seen, a more informative way of expressing the result. You will see, from reading medical journals nowadays, that p values are routinely and extensively quoted in statistical analyses.

Because computers remove the computational chore from statistical work, it is an easy matter to use them to carry out extensive analyses, repeated analyses and thorough analyses. What is meant under this last category is, for example, the proper checking of an analysis. An example of this would be the checking of residuals after regression analysis. This is a step which is all too easily overlooked in the analysis, but which is a vital part of the full analysis. At the beginning of an analysis, statistical computer packages can (and should) be used as very valuable tools in looking at the data and getting a thoroughly good feel for the data. (This is important in the sense that one then knows what to expect from a formal analysis of the data and hence it can lead to better confidence in the results when they are obtained.) Statistical reports of medical data seem to have regrettably few graphs in them (summaries of the data are more often tabulated), but this should not prevent the person carrying out the analysis from looking at as many graphs of the data as possible on the computer screen, even if most of them will not be used in the final report. For example, the starting point in the analysis of data from a clinical trial is often to scan profiles over time of key efficacy variables for all the patients in the trial.

In summary, statistical computer packages constitute a very powerful and useful tool in modern statistical analysis, and make possible many things that could not be contemplated some years ago. They should, however, be used with extreme caution and much thought, and with a readiness always to supplement them with expert advice when necessary.

NOTE

You have done well to complete this programme, particularly if you have not sneaked a look at the answers before attempting to solve the frames yourself.

This is the programmed part of the book concluded. To follow, we have the answers to the practical examples and a test for those who choose to pit their wits and to gain further practice in what they have learnt.

Primarily, you should now be able to understand what most simple statistical jargon is about. You should also be able to perform simple tests for yourself.

If people did not vary, we could add and subtract information about them as if they were no more than a problem in simple arithmetic. Fortunately, people not only look different, they think differently and they act differently. G. K. Chesterton had it neatly summed up when he said that, 'Man is a biped, but fifty men are not a centipede'.

Statistics, in terms of medical research, is only the application of numerical common sense to data which are subject to variation, about health and disease. In fact it is more a question of collecting the right data to collate than of prescribing the most appropriate mathematical formulae. It is no good applying a healthy significance test to a sample of people who are sick in terms of the research design. Always ask yourself whether the control group is correctly chosen, whether the comparison is meaningful in terms of the stated purpose of the work, etc. Keep your eyes open – you will not be bored. In the medical profession statistics is often used as a drunken man uses a lamp-post – for support rather than illumination. A lot of the medical literature deals with groups of people who vary. Medical applications of statistics can be far-reaching but often this particular union turns out to be an unholy alliance rather than a happy marriage.

We despise a shoddy diagnosis, and rightly so. How can we tolerate, in print (or anywhere else for that matter) incorrect statistics leading to incorrect conclusions? Some may choose to dismiss this criticism with a Shakespearean shrug, 'What is a lie? 'Tis but the truth in masquerade'. Yet one does not have to have a tremendously deep mathematical know-how to help us salvage our damaged reputation.

How does one select the correct research design and collect the correct data to analyse? The first requirement has to be a clear-cut honesty, not only with those people likely to read the work but, most important of all, with oneself. Each method of tracking a research problem leads to different results and different conclusions. It is therefore necessary to be selective in the choice of methodology. To a large extent, we can be wise by being uncomplicated, by remaining simple.

We can, for example, spell out exactly what it is we are trying to achieve, define our medical terms, decide at the beginning whether we want to compare our results with another worker's, and, if so, we can establish the same methodology. We can define the population, and choose reliable samples and reliable and motivated research assistants (the fewer the better).

The analysis is only one facet of the statistical scene. It must be emphasised that although the conclusions may be interesting, their validity is of fundamental importance.

Answers to practical examples

2.23 Country of origin of doctors practising in a newly developed African country.

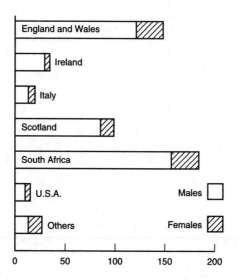

3.30

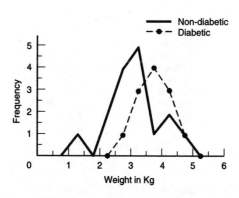

Birth-weight of children of diabetic and non-diabetic mothers.

5.29 For example:

	x	$(x - \bar{x})$	$(x - \bar{x})^2$	x	(x^2)
1	2	−3	9	2	4
2	4	−1	1	4	16
3	5	0	0	5	25
4	3	−2	4	3	9
5	6	+1	1	6	36
6	9	+4	16	9	81
7	9	+4	16	9	81
8	1	−4	16	1	1
9	0	−5	25	0	0
10	11	+6	36	11	121

$$\Sigma(x) = 50 \quad \Sigma(x - \bar{x}) = 0 \quad \Sigma(x - \bar{x})^2 = 124 \quad \Sigma(x) = 50 \quad \Sigma(x^2) = 374$$
$$\bar{x} = 5$$

$$\therefore \frac{\Sigma(x - \bar{x})^2}{n - 1} = \frac{124}{9} = 13\frac{7}{9}$$

$$\frac{\Sigma(x^2) - \frac{(\Sigma x)^2}{n}}{n - 1} = \frac{374 - \frac{50^2}{10}}{9}$$

$$= \frac{374 - 250}{9} = \frac{124}{9} = 13\frac{7}{9}$$

7.45

Frame 3.1		Frame 3.5	
x	x^2	x	x^2
2.92	8.5264	1.47	2.1609
3.23	10.4329	2.24	5.0176
3.23	10.4329	2.27	5.1529
3.46	11.9716	2.84	8.0656
3.71	13.7641	2.94	8.6436
3.91	15.2881	2.95	8.7025
3.91	15.2881	2.95	8.7025
3.91	15.2881	3.01	9.0601
4.05	16.4025	3.09	9.5481
4.14	17.1396	3.15	9.9225
4.28	18.3184	3.40	11.5600
4.82	23.2324	3.43	11.7649
		3.60	12.9600
		4.22	17.8084
		4.25	18.0625
		4.59	21.0681
$\Sigma(x) = 45.57$	$\Sigma(x^2) = 176.0851$	$\Sigma(x) = 50.40$	$\Sigma(x^2) = 168.2002$
$n = 12$		$n = 16$	
$\bar{x} = 3.798$		$\bar{x} = 3.150$	

7.45 *cont'd*

$$s^2 = \frac{176.0851 - \frac{(45.57)^2}{12}}{11}$$
$$= 0.2757$$
$$\therefore s = 0.525$$

$$s^2 = \frac{168.2002 - \frac{(50.40)^2}{16}}{15}$$
$$= 0.6293$$
$$\therefore s = 0.793$$

9.43 (1) Scatter diagram

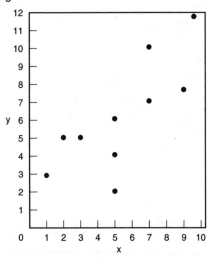

(2) Estimate of the correlation coefficient could be $+0.8$.

(3) Calculation of r:

x	y	x^2	y^2	xy
1	3	1	9	3
2	5	4	25	10
3	5	9	25	15
5	2	25	4	10
5	4	25	16	20
5	6	25	36	30
7	7	49	49	49
7	10	49	100	70
9	8	81	64	72
10	12	100	144	120
$\Sigma(x) = 54$	$\Sigma(y) = 62$	$\Sigma(x^2) = 368$	$\Sigma(y^2) = 472$	$\Sigma(xy) = 399$

9.43 *cont'd*
$n = 10$

$$r = \frac{\Sigma(xy) - \dfrac{(\Sigma x)(\Sigma y)}{n}}{\sqrt{\left[\Sigma(x^2) - \dfrac{(\Sigma x)^2}{n}\right]\left[\Sigma(y^2) - \dfrac{(\Sigma y)^2}{n}\right]}}$$

$$\therefore r = \frac{399 - \dfrac{54 \times 62}{10}}{\sqrt{\left[368 - \dfrac{(54)^2}{10}\right]\left[472 - \dfrac{(62)^2}{10}\right]}}$$

$$= \frac{399 - 334.8}{\sqrt{(368 - 291.6)(472 - 384.4)}}$$

$$= \frac{64.2}{\sqrt{(76.4)(87.6)}} = \frac{64.2}{\sqrt{6692.64}} = \frac{64.2}{81.809}$$

$$= +0.78$$

(4)   Calculation of ρ:

x	y	Ranked x	Ranked y	d	d^2
1	3	10	9	$+1$	1
2	5	9	$6\frac{1}{2}$	$+2\frac{1}{2}$	$6\frac{1}{4}$
3	5	8	$6\frac{1}{2}$	$+1\frac{1}{2}$	$2\frac{1}{4}$
5	2	6	10	-4	16
5	4	6	8	-2	4
5	6	6	5	$+1$	1
7	7	$3\frac{1}{2}$	4	$-\frac{1}{2}$	$\frac{1}{4}$
7	10	$3\frac{1}{2}$	2	$+1\frac{1}{2}$	$2\frac{1}{4}$
9	8	2	3	-1	1
10	12	1	1	0	0
		Sum to 55	Sum to 55	$\Sigma(d) = 0$	$\Sigma(d^2) = 34$

$n = 10$

$$\rho = 1 - \frac{6\Sigma d^2}{n(n^2 - 1)}$$

$$\therefore \rho = 1 - \frac{6 \times 34}{10 \times 99}$$

$$= 1 - \frac{34}{165}$$

$$= +0.79$$

9.43 *cont'd*

$\therefore r = +0.78$ and $\rho = +0.79$

which are approximately the same.

Of course r is the more accurate estimate as it uses all the information.

11.61 You ought to have thought of most of the following points:

1) **Definition of the population**
   The doctor must fully and exhaustively define his population so that it is absolutely clear who are to be included and excluded. For example is he running his trials on any adults in the population, or only on females? How is he going to define overweight? Is he going to attempt to exclude people with renal or hormonal disease and, if so, how?

2) **Factors affecting precision**
   Is he going to weigh patients dressed only in a gown provided at the time? At what time of day will he weigh the subjects? What decisions is he going to make about diet? Over what period of time will he measure the decrease in weight, and how often will he weigh the subjects? How many subjects will he include? (Actually, he would need to know more than we are able to cover in this book to be able to work out what this should be. He would need to have some idea of the minimum difference in weight changes that would be of interest, and also what the likely variability in the weights is.)

3) **Factors affecting bias**
   The trial will fortunately be prospective and objective. Random samples must be selected. If the patients are allocated numbers consecutively as they enter the trial the numbers can previously have been assigned to the different treatments using tables of random numbers. Will any stratification be necessary to take account of, for example, different ethnic groups? One group will be the control group on a placebo.

4) **Other factors**
   Check the results will be analysable before starting (you will learn one test which is suitable soon). Decide before starting what will be done with patients who drop out of the trials. Decide what records of drug side-effects must be kept and what will be done with them.

15.62 This is a one-tailed test as the surgeon's wife was only interested in the physician's prowess at tossing tails.

The answer depends on the significance level. We see this as follows:

The probability of tossing 1 tail is $\dfrac{1}{2} = 0.5$

15.62 *cont'd*

The probability of tossing 2 tails is $\left(\dfrac{1}{2}\right)^2 = 0.25$

The probability of tossing 3 tails is $\left(\dfrac{1}{2}\right)^3 = 0.125$

The probability of tossing 4 tails is $\left(\dfrac{1}{2}\right)^4 = 0.0625$

The probability of tossing 5 tails is $\left(\dfrac{1}{2}\right)^5 = 0.03125$

Hence, considering the 0.05 significance level, p is less than 0.05 at 5 throws and she should have persuaded her husband to stop then.

However, for the significance level of 0.01, p only becomes less than this value at the seventh throw.

Similarly, in a drug trial if all 5 patients in the trial prefer drug A, then the result is significant at the 0.05 level. With a slightly larger group of patients in a trial, if all 7 prefer A and none B, this is significant at the 0.01 level.

16.51 The Null Hypothesis states that there is no significant difference. The alternative is that B_{12} increases weight gain.

Calculated $z = \dfrac{\bar{x}_1 - \bar{x}_2}{\sqrt{\dfrac{s_1^2}{n_1} + \dfrac{s_2^2}{n_2}}}$

$$\therefore z = \dfrac{156 - 148}{\sqrt{\dfrac{37^2}{50} + \dfrac{40^2}{50}}}$$

$$= \dfrac{8}{\sqrt{\dfrac{2969}{50}}} = \dfrac{8}{7.706} = 1.04$$

This is a one-tailed test.

The significant (critical) z values are 1.64 (0.05) and 2.33 (0.01). The calculated z value is less than these significant values (critical values) of z and hence p is greater than the significance levels:

$$p > 0.05$$

Therefore either B_{12} does not increase the weight gain or there is insufficient evidence that it does so.

17.62 The Null Hypothesis states that there is no significant difference.

It is a one-tailed test.

$\bar{x}_1$ for diabetic mothers is 3.798.

$n_1 = 12$

$\bar{x}_2$ for non-diabetic mothers is 3.150.

$n_2 = 16$

$\therefore f = n_1 + n_2 - 2 = 26$

$t = \dfrac{\bar{x}_1 - \bar{x}_2}{s\sqrt{\dfrac{1}{n_1} + \dfrac{1}{n_2}}}$, assuming equal variance for diabetic and non-diabetic mothers,

where $s^2 = \dfrac{(\Sigma x_1^2) - \dfrac{(\Sigma x_1)^2}{n_1} + \Sigma (x_2^2) - \dfrac{(\Sigma x_2)^2}{n_2}}{n_1 + n_2 - 2}$

$= \dfrac{(176.0851 - 173.0521) + (168.2002 - 158.7600)}{26}$

$= \dfrac{12.4732}{26} = 0.4797$

$\therefore s = 0.6926$

$\therefore t = \dfrac{3.798 - 3.150}{0.6926\sqrt{\dfrac{1}{12} + \dfrac{1}{16}}} = \dfrac{0.648}{0.2645} = 2.45$

The tabulated values of t with $f = 26$ for a one-tailed test are 1.706 for a significance level of 0.05 and 2.479 for the 0.01 significance level.
$\therefore 0.05 > p > 0.01$

Hence, the conclusion is that the mean birth-weight of children of diabetic mothers is significantly bigger than the mean birth-weight of children of mothers in the control group at the 0.05 significance level, but not at the 0.01 level (although almost so at this level too, since 2.45 is close to 2.479).

17.63 **Question 1**
The Null Hypothesis is that there is no difference in caecal length between the sexes, and the Alternative Hypothesis is that there is a difference. More specifically, these hypotheses should be stated in terms of the mean lengths, so we have:

Null Hypothesis: $\mu_1 = \mu_2$,

Alternative Hypothesis: $\mu_1 \neq \mu_2$,

σ unknown, $n < 30$, μ unknown

17.63 *cont'd*

$$\therefore \text{Use } t = \frac{\bar{x}_1 - \bar{x}_2}{s\sqrt{\dfrac{1}{n_1} + \dfrac{1}{n_2}}} \text{ where } s^2 = \frac{\Sigma(x_1 - \bar{x}_1)^2 + \Sigma(x_2 - \bar{x}_2)^2}{n_1 + n_2 - 2}$$

$\bar{x}_1 = 14.8;\ \bar{x}_2 = 13.7;\ s^2 = 0.81;\ n_1 = 25;\ n_2 = 20$

$$\therefore \text{Calculated } t = \frac{14.8 - 13.7}{0.9\sqrt{\dfrac{1}{25} + \dfrac{1}{20}}} = \frac{1.1}{0.27} \simeq 4$$

$f = n_1 + n_2 - 2 = 43$ which is not shown in the t tables in this book. (If $f = 29$ or bigger the value of t does not change much and we use the bottom line – remember, when f is very large, the t values are the same as the normal-distribution z values.)

This is a two-tailed test.

Significant (critical) $t = 1.960$ (0.05) or 2.576 (0.01) (using the normal distribution values – the t values with 40 degrees of freedom are 2.021 and 2.704 respectively).

$\therefore$ The calculated value of $t >$ significant t (at both these levels).

There is a significant difference between the results ($p < 0.01$). (If $p < 0.01$, as here, we often say that the difference is highly significant.)

More specifically we can say that there is a highly significant difference ($p < 0.01$) between the mean caecal lengths, comparing the sexes.

Question 2

The Null Hypothesis is that there is no difference in the amount that the two types of patients eat, and the Alternative Hypothesis is that there is a difference. More specifically:

Null Hypothesis: $\mu = 0$,
Alternative Hypothesis: $\mu > 0$,
where μ is now the mean paired difference (amount eaten by cancer patient minus amount eaten by paired non-cancer patient).

σ unknown, $n < 30$, paired results (matched)

$$\therefore \text{Use } t = \frac{\bar{x} - \mu}{\dfrac{s}{\sqrt{n}}} \text{ on the paired results.}$$

$\bar{x} = 180;\ s = 450;\ n = 25;\ \mu = 0$

$$\therefore t = \frac{180 - 0}{\dfrac{450}{\sqrt{25}}} = 2$$

This is a one-tailed test with $f = 24$.

$\therefore$ Significant $t = 1.711$ (0.05) and 2.492 (0.01) (from the table).

17.63   Question 2 *cont'd*

These results can be summarised as $0.05 > p > 0.01$.

People with cancer of the stomach on average ate significantly more than other patients at the 0.05 (5%) significance level, but not at the 0.01 (1%) significance level.

Question 3

The Null Hypothesis is that there is no difference in blood alcohol levels between those who had been involved in car accidents and those who had not, and the Alternative Hypothesis is that the blood alcohol level in drivers who had car accidents is higher. More specifically:

Null Hypothesis: $\mu_1 = \mu_2$,
Alternative Hypothesis: $\mu_1 > \mu_2$,
where μ_1 corresponds to drivers who had a car accident and μ_2 to those who did not.

σ unknown, $n > 30$, μ unknown

$$\therefore z = \frac{\bar{x}_1 - \bar{x}_2}{\sqrt{\dfrac{s_1^2}{n_1} + \dfrac{s_2^2}{n_2}}}$$

(This is an approximation, allowable because of the large sample size.)

$\bar{x}_1 = 2.42$; $\bar{x}_2 = 2.24$; $s_1^2 = 0.39$; $s_2^2 = 0.25$

$n_1 = 100$; $n_2 = 100$

$$\therefore \text{Calculated } z = \frac{2.42 - 2.24}{\sqrt{\dfrac{0.39}{100} + \dfrac{0.25}{100}}} = \frac{0.18}{0.08} = 2.25$$

This is a one-tailed test.

$\therefore$ Significant (critical) $z = 1.645$ (0.05) or 2.326 (0.01)

i.e. $0.05 > p > 0.01$

At the 0.05 level you accept that the rate of accidents was significantly affected by the alcohol level but at the 0.01 level you conclude that either there is no effect or that there is insufficient evidence.

If we used a t test, adopting the approach that whenever σ is unknown, we estimate it by s, and use t, we would have:

$$t = \frac{\bar{x}_1 - \bar{x}_2}{s\sqrt{\dfrac{1}{n_1} + \dfrac{1}{n_2}}}, \text{ assuming equal variances amongst drivers who had a}$$

car accident and those who did not,

$$\text{where } s^2 = \frac{(n_1 - 1)s_1^2 + (n_2 - 1)s_2^2}{n_1 + n_2 - 2},$$

17.63   *cont'd*

$$so\ s^2 = \frac{(99 \times 0.39) + (99 \times 0.25)}{198}$$

$$= \frac{0.64}{2} = 0.32$$

Hence $s = 0.5657$

Then $t = \dfrac{2.42 - 2.24}{0.5657\sqrt{\dfrac{1}{100} + \dfrac{1}{100}}} = \dfrac{0.18}{0.0800}$

$$= 2.25$$

The rest follows as before.

18.20   The Null Hypothesis is that there is no real correlation, i.e. that the correlation is zero. The Alternative Hypothesis is that there is real correlation, i.e. that the correlation is different from zero. The corresponding test is two-tailed.

Tabulated $t\,(f = 8)$ is 2.306 (0.05) or 3.355 (0.01).

Calculated $t = \dfrac{0.78\sqrt{8}}{\sqrt{(1 - 0.78^2)}} = \dfrac{0.78 \times 2.828}{\sqrt{(1 - 0.608)}} = \dfrac{2.206}{0.626}$

$$= 3.5$$

Calculated t is bigger than significant (critical) t at both levels ($p < 0.01$). The conclusion is that there is evidence of a real correlation between erythrocyte sedimentation rate and number of leucocytes.

These results may well be summarised in a medical journal as follows:

'$r = +0.78$. This is evidence of real correlation ($t = 3.5$, $p < 0.01$).'
(0.79 may be substituted for ρ to reach the same conclusion.)

20.68   The Null Hypothesis is that any difference in distribution over sites of benign and malignant cerebral tumours is due entirely to chance, or that there is no association between site of tumour and type of tumour. The Alternative Hypothesis is that there is association between the site and type of the cerebral tumours.
The corresponding test is one-tailed.

Using the fact that: Expected result $= \dfrac{\text{Row total} \times \text{Column total}}{\text{Grand total}}$

the contingency table for expected values becomes:

20.68   *cont'd*

	Benign	Malignant	
Frontal lobe	26.67	13.33	40
Temporal lobe	20.00	10.00	30
Other lobes	53.33	26.67	80
	100	50	150

No expected result is less than 5 so we can calculate $\chi^2 = \sum \dfrac{(O - E)^2}{E}$.

O	E	$O - E$	$(O - E)^2$	$\dfrac{(O - E)^2}{E}$
21	26.67	−5.67	32.15	1.21
28	20.00	+8.00	64.00	3.20
51	53.33	−2.33	5.43	0.10
19	13.33	+5.67	32.15	2.41
2	10.00	−8.00	64.00	6.40
29	26.67	+2.33	5.43	0.20
				13.52

$$\therefore \sum \frac{(O - E)^2}{E} = 13.5$$

The tabulated value of χ^2 $(f = (r - 1)(c - 1) = 2) = 5.991$ for a significance level of 0.05 and 9.210 for a significance level of 0.01. The calculated χ^2 is greater than both these tabulated values of χ^2. The conclusion is therefore that there is an association between the type and the site of cerebral tumours ($p < 0.01$).

How much have you learnt?

This is to test your knowledge – the answers are given at the end of the test.

1. (a) Give an example of continuous quantitative data.

   (b) Give an example of discrete quantitative data.

   (c) Give an example of qualitative data.

   (d) Give two reasons why these distinctions are important in statistics.

2. Of 200 births in the Lady Chatterley's Maternity Home last year, 90 were females.
   (a) What was the ratio of males to females?
   (b) What was the proportion of females?
   (c) What was the percentage of females?

3. Is

   $$\frac{\text{the number of sailors killed at Trafalgar}}{\text{the number of sailors involved at Trafalgar}}$$

   a ratio, a rate, a proportion or a percentage?

4. Make a rough sketch of
   (a) a histogram, and
   (b) a pie diagram.

5. When would you use a frequency polygon to present data?

6. The diagram below represents a distribution of data.
   (a) What is it called?
   (b) Mark in the position of the mean.
   (c) What is the length of AB called?
       (B is a point of inflection.)

6.   *cont'd*

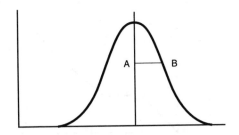

7.   What is the difference between $\Sigma(x^2)$ and $(\Sigma x)^2$?

8.   Calculate the mean, median and mode of the following distribution:
      1, 2, 2, 2, 3, 5, 5, 6, 6, 18.

9.   Why is the mean a better (in some sense) measure of the middle than either the median or the mode?

10.   Why is the sum of the deviations from the mean not used as a measure of variation?

11. Σ means 'the sum of'.
      x is an observed result.
      $\bar{x}$ is the mean.
      s is the standard deviation.
      n is the number of results.

      What is wrong with the following equation?

      $$s = \frac{\Sigma(x - \bar{x})^2}{n - 1}$$

12.   The variance of 1, 2, 3, 3, 4, 5 is 2.
      What is the value of the standard deviation?
      What is the value of the range?

13.   Which is the better measure of variation, the range or the standard deviation?
      Why?

14.   Why is this not a good diagram?

14.   *cont'd*

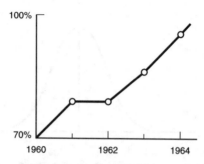

Percentage Pass rate in Anatomy at a particular Medical School (1960–64 inclusive)

15.   What do you understand by 'correlation'?

16.   What are the maximum and minimum numerical values of a correlation coefficient? What is the value when there is no correlation?

17.   The diagram below shows corresponding values for x and y. What is the value of the correlation coefficient here?

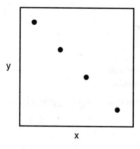

18.   What is the main difference between Pearson's and Spearman's correlation coefficients?

19. ρ is Spearman's correlation coefficient:

$$\rho = 1 - \frac{6\Sigma d^2}{n(n^2 - 1)}.$$

n is the number of pairs of results. What does d represent?

20. s is a statistic and σ is a parameter and both represent the standard deviation. What is the difference in the meaning of these two symbols?

21. What do you understand by the term 'bias'? What method would you use to reduce bias?

22. Precision can be used to describe how close various estimates of a population mean are to each other. How would you improve the precision of a sample?

23. You are interested in the I.Q.'s of this year's 1st year medical students at a particular university as opposed to students in other faculties. Define your control group exactly.

24. You are told that the probability of some event equals one. What does this mean?

25. (a) What is the probability of throwing a 2 or a 6 with a fair die?
    (b) What is the probability of throwing a 2 and a 6 with two dice?

26. What type of sampling distribution is this?

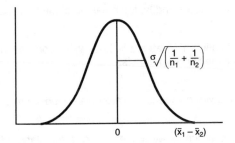

27. There are many possible normal distributions. These can be standardised to a single normal distribution called the *standard* normal distribution (shown below). Label the arrows.

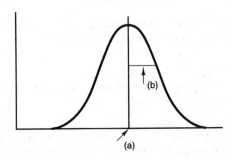

28.   What is the value of z, the standard normal deviate, corresponding to the number 6 in this diagram?

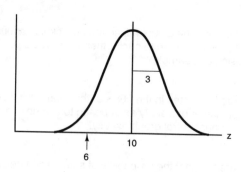

29.   (a) What is the special name for the standard deviation of the sampling distribution of the mean?
        (b) How is it related to the population standard deviation?

30.   What is the use of a significance level?

31.   What do you understand by the meaning of the term 'Null Hypothesis'?

32.   An article in a journal states '$p > 0.05$'. What conclusion would you draw about the Null Hypothesis?

33.   What makes you decide to use a one- as opposed to a two-tailed test?

34.   Give the difference between the uses of z, the standard normal deviate, and Student's t (t test) with respect to:
        (a) the sample size,
        (b) s^2 and σ^2,
        (c) the number of degrees of freedom, f.

35.   If you know the formula for calculating s^2 how can you use it to calculate the number of degrees of freedom?

36.   Look at page 279.
        What is the significant (critical) value of t at the 5% significance level (two-tailed test) where $f = 3$?

37.   What does a coefficient of correlation between two variables tell you about the magnitude of the regression coefficient corresponding to the line of regression of one on the other?

38. A regression line is fitted to a set of data. What are the residuals?

39. In a simple linear regression there are two types of variable. One is called the dependent variable. What is the other called?

40. In a regression analysis, what assumptions should hold for the residuals?

41. What conditions have to be satisfied for the application of χ^2 (chi-squared)?

42. Is a χ^2 distribution symmetric?

43. This is a 2 × 2 contingency table of observed results:

	A	Not A	
B	10	20	30
Not B	30	40	70
	40	60	100

(a) Complete the equivalent expected table:

	A	Not A
B		
Not B		

(b) How many degrees of freedom are there in this table?

44. Look at page 280. The calculated value of χ^2 (chi-squared) with 11 degrees of freedom is 18.002. What is your conclusion:
(a) in a one-tailed test with the significance level 0.05?
(b) in a two-tailed test with the significance level 0.01?

45. What does a p value of 0.99 probably mean in a χ^2 test?

46. When would you consider using a nonparametric test?

47. If the failure of distributional assumptions leads you to consider using a nonparametric test, what alternative approach might you consider?

48. To what types of Student's *t* tests do (a) the Mann–Whitney *U* test, and (b) the Wilcoxon matched-pairs signed-rank test correspond?

49. An analysis is carried out using a statistical package. In fact, the underlying assumptions for the analysis are not satisfied. But the package produces all the output that you expect, with neatly printed results. So all is well after all. True or false?

ANSWERS TO TEST

1.   (a) Haemoglobin level. Bladder volume.
       (b) Pain score, on a 1 to 5 rating scale. Number of decayed teeth.
       (c) Sex. Blood groups.
       (d) The different types of data are presented differently and are subjected to different tests.

2.   (a) 110 : 90, or 11 : 9

       (b) $\dfrac{90}{200}$ or $\dfrac{9}{20}$

       (c) 45%

3.   Proportion

4.

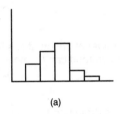

(a)

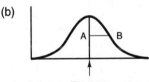

(b)

5.   When the data are quantitative, especially when two sets of data are to be illustrated on the same diagram.

6.   (a) The normal distribution

       (b)

The mean

       (c) The standard deviation

7. $\Sigma(x^2)$ is the sum of the numbers already squared.
       $(\Sigma x)^2$ is the square of the numbers already summed.

8. The mean   = 5
   The median = 4
   The mode   = 2

9. It uses all the information (and is amenable to mathematical manipulation in, for example, significance tests).

10. It always equals zero.

11. $s^2 = \dfrac{\Sigma(x - \bar{x})^2}{n - 1}$ or $s = \sqrt{\dfrac{\Sigma(x - \bar{x})^2}{n - 1}}$

12. The standard deviation = $\sqrt{2}$
    The range   = 4

13. The standard deviation (unless the number of observations is very small), because it uses all the information (and can be more easily used further in significance tests).

14. The zero is suppressed and the line is extrapolated.

15. A measure of linear association

16. The maximum value   = +1
    The minimum value   = −1
    When there is no correlation the value   = 0

17. −1

18. Pearson's uses the actual results and Spearman's uses the ranks.

19. d is the difference between ranks.

20. s is the standard deviation in a sample, σ is the standard deviation in the population.

21. Bias is the off-target effect of statistics. Randomisation and 'blind' sampling are examples.

22.   Increase its size

23.   A random sample of I.Q.'s of this year's 1st year students in other faculties at the university.

24.   It is inevitable.

25.   a) $\dfrac{1}{3}$ b) $\dfrac{2}{36}$ or $\dfrac{1}{18}$

26.   The distribution of the differences between two sample means

27.   (a) The mean = 0   (b) The standard deviation = 1

28. $-1^{1}/_{3}$

29.   The standard error of the mean.
      It equals the population standard deviation divided by $\sqrt{n}$.

30.   It enables decisions to be made.

31.   It is a precise statement against which to test observed results.

32.   It is either true or there is as yet insufficient evidence to reject it at the 0.05 (5%) significance level.

33.   The Alternative Hypothesis is concerned with outcomes in one direction only.

34. t is used
      (a) with small samples (say n less than 30) – and, strictly speaking, even with larger samples when σ is unknown;
      (b) with s^{2}; and
      (c) depends on the number of degrees of freedom, f.

      z is used
      (a) with large samples (say n at least as large as 30) as an approximation and with smaller samples only if σ^2 is known.
      (b) It can be used with σ^2, or with s^2 as an approximation in large samples.
      (c) It does not depend on the number of degrees of freedom.

35. The number of degrees of freedom equals the denominator.

36. 3.182

37. Nothing

38. The differences between the fitted values and the observed values, in the direction of the dependent variable

39. Independent, or regressor, variable

40. They should have independent normal distributions with zero mean and constant variance.

41. The samples are random.
    The data are qualitative.
    There is ideally no expected value less than 5 (or very few of them).

42. In general, no – in fact when the associated number of degrees of freedom is small, it is highly skewed (i.e. highly asymmetric). Only when the number of degrees of freedom is very large is the χ^2 distribution approximated by the normal distribution, and hence nearly symmetric.

43. (a)

	A	Not A	
B	12	18	30
Not B	28	42	70
	40	60	100

(b) $f = 1$

44. (a) Reject the Null Hypothesis, accept the Alternative.

    (b) Either the Null Hypothesis is true or there is insufficient evidence to reject it.

45. Suspect cheating.

46. When the underlying assumptions, particularly distributional, for a classical parametric test do not hold.

47. Transform the data so that the distributional assumptions hold and then use the appropriate parametric test.

48. (a) A two-sample t-test for the difference between two means.
   (b) A matched-pairs t-test (for the difference of a mean difference from zero).

49. False! Beware of obtaining an analysis from the computer which looks correct because it is nicely printed out. If rubbish goes in (e.g. applying an inappropriate analysis – possibly because of the failure of underlying assumptions – to a set of data), rubbish will come out, however neat it looks!

TABLES

PEARSON'S CORRELATION COEFFICIENT

$$r = \frac{\Sigma(xy) - \dfrac{\Sigma(x)\,\Sigma(y)}{n}}{\sqrt{\left[\Sigma(x^2) - \dfrac{(\Sigma x)^2}{n}\right]\left[\Sigma(y^2) - \dfrac{(\Sigma y)^2}{n}\right]}}$$

SPEARMAN'S RANK-ORDER CORRELATION COEFFICIENT

$$\rho = 1 - \frac{6\Sigma(d^2)}{n(n^2 - 1)}$$

THE NORMAL DISTRIBUTION

p	0.10	0.05	0.02	0.01
z	1.645	1.960	2.326	2.576

CRITICAL VALUES FOR THE WILCOXON SIGNED-RANK TEST

n	$\alpha_1=$ 5% $\alpha_2=$ 10%	$2\frac{1}{2}$% 5%	1% 2%	$\frac{1}{2}$% 1%	n	$\alpha_1=$ 5% $\alpha_2=$ 10%	$2\frac{1}{2}$% 5%	1% 2%	$\frac{1}{2}$% 1%
1	–	–	–	–	26	110	98	84	75
2	–	–	–	–	27	119	107	92	83
3	–	–	–	–	28	130	116	101	91
4	–	–	–	–	29	140	126	110	100
5	0	–	–	–	30	151	137	120	109
6	2	0	–	–	31	163	147	130	118
7	3	2	0	–	32	175	159	140	128
8	5	3	1	0	33	187	170	151	138
9	8	5	3	1	34	200	182	162	148
10	10	8	5	3	35	213	195	173	159
11	13	10	7	5	36	227	208	185	171
12	17	13	9	7	37	241	221	198	182
13	21	17	12	9	38	256	235	211	194
14	25	21	15	12	39	271	249	224	207
15	30	25	19	15	40	286	264	238	220
16	35	29	23	19	41	302	279	252	233
17	41	34	27	23	42	319	294	266	247
18	47	40	32	27	43	336	310	281	261
19	53	46	37	32	44	353	327	296	276
20	60	52	43	37	45	371	343	312	291
21	67	58	49	42	46	389	361	328	307
22	75	65	55	48	47	407	378	345	322
23	83	73	62	54	48	426	396	362	339
24	91	81	69	61	49	446	415	379	355
25	100	89	76	68	50	466	434	397	373

CRITICAL VALUES FOR THE MANN–WHITNEY TEST

n_1	n_2	$\alpha_1=$ 5% $\alpha_2=$ 10%	2½% 5%	1% 2%	½% 1%	n_1	n_2	$\alpha_1=$ 5% $\alpha_2=$ 10%	2½% 5%	1% 2%	½% 1%
2	2	–	–	–	–	4	17	15	11	8	6
2	3	–	–	–	–	4	18	16	12	9	6
2	4	–	–	–	–	4	19	17	13	9	7
2	5	0	–	–	–	4	20	18	14	10	8
2	6	0	–	–	–						
2	7	0	–	–	–	5	5	4	2	1	0
2	8	1	0	–	–	5	6	5	3	2	1
2	9	1	0	–	–	5	7	6	5	3	1
2	10	1	0	–	–	5	8	8	6	4	2
2	11	1	0	–	–	5	9	9	7	5	3
2	12	2	1	–	–	5	10	11	8	6	4
2	13	2	1	0	–	5	11	12	9	7	5
2	14	3	1	0	–	5	12	13	11	8	6
2	15	3	1	0	–	5	13	15	12	9	7
2	16	3	1	0	–	5	14	16	13	10	7
2	17	3	2	0	–	5	15	18	14	11	8
2	18	4	2	0	–	5	16	19	15	12	9
2	19	4	2	1	0	5	17	20	17	13	10
2	20	4	2	1	0	5	18	22	18	14	11
						5	19	23	19	15	12
3	3	0	–	–	–	5	20	25	20	16	13
3	4	0	–	–	–						
3	5	1	0	–	–	6	6	7	5	3	2
3	6	2	1	–	–	6	7	8	6	4	3
3	7	2	1	0	–	6	8	10	8	6	4
3	8	3	2	0	–	6	9	12	10	7	5
3	9	4	2	1	0	6	10	14	11	8	6
3	10	4	3	1	0	6	11	16	13	9	7
3	11	5	3	1	0	6	12	17	14	11	9
3	12	5	4	2	1	6	13	19	16	12	10
3	13	6	4	2	1	6	14	21	17	13	11
3	14	7	5	2	1	6	15	23	19	15	12
3	15	7	5	3	2	6	16	25	21	16	13
3	16	8	6	3	2	6	17	26	22	18	15
3	17	9	6	4	2	6	18	28	24	19	16
3	18	9	7	4	2	6	19	30	25	20	17
3	19	10	7	4	3	6	20	32	27	22	18
3	20	11	8	5	3						
						7	7	11	8	6	4
4	4	1	0	–	–	7	8	13	10	7	6
4	5	2	1	0	–	7	9	15	12	9	7
4	6	3	2	1	0	7	10	17	14	11	9
4	7	4	3	1	0	7	11	19	16	12	10
4	8	5	4	2	1	7	12	21	18	14	12
4	9	6	4	3	1	7	13	24	20	16	13
4	10	7	5	3	2	7	14	26	22	17	15
4	11	8	6	4	2	7	15	28	24	19	16
4	12	9	7	5	3	7	16	30	26	21	18
4	13	10	8	5	3	7	17	33	28	23	19
4	14	11	9	6	4	7	18	35	30	24	21
4	15	12	10	7	5	7	19	37	32	26	22
4	16	14	11	7	5	7	20	39	34	28	24

continued

n_1	n_2	$\alpha_1 =$ 5% $\alpha_2 =$ 10%	2½% 5%	1% 2%	½% 1%	n_1	n_2	$\alpha_1 =$ 5% $\alpha_2 =$ 10%	2½% 5%	1% 2%	½% 1%
8	8	15	13	9	7	12	12	42	37	31	27
8	9	18	15	11	9	12	13	47	41	35	31
8	10	20	17	13	11	12	14	51	45	38	34
8	11	23	19	15	13	12	15	55	49	42	37
8	12	26	22	17	15	12	16	60	53	46	41
8	13	28	24	20	17	12	17	64	57	49	44
8	14	31	26	22	18	12	18	68	61	53	47
8	15	33	29	24	20	12	19	72	65	56	51
8	16	36	31	26	22	12	20	77	69	60	54
8	17	39	34	28	24						
8	18	41	36	30	26	13	13	51	45	39	34
8	19	44	38	32	28	13	14	56	50	43	38
8	20	47	41	34	30	13	15	61	54	47	42
						13	16	65	59	51	45
9	9	21	17	14	11	13	17	70	63	55	49
9	10	24	20	16	13	13	18	75	67	59	53
9	11	27	23	18	16	13	19	80	72	63	57
9	12	30	26	21	18	13	20	84	76	67	60
9	13	33	28	23	20						
9	14	36	31	26	22	14	14	61	55	47	42
9	15	39	34	28	24	14	15	66	59	51	46
9	16	42	37	31	27	14	16	71	64	56	50
9	17	45	39	33	29	14	17	77	69	60	54
9	18	48	42	36	31	14	18	82	74	65	58
9	19	51	45	38	33	14	19	87	78	60	63
9	20	54	48	40	36	14	20	92	83	73	67
10	10	27	23	19	16	15	15	72	64	56	51
10	11	31	26	22	18	15	16	77	70	61	55
10	12	34	29	24	21	15	17	83	75	66	60
10	13	37	33	27	24	15	18	88	80	70	64
10	14	41	36	30	26	15	19	94	85	75	69
10	15	44	39	33	29	15	20	100	90	80	73
10	16	48	42	36	31						
10	17	51	45	38	34	16	16	83	75	66	60
10	18	55	48	41	37	16	17	89	81	71	65
10	19	58	52	44	39	16	18	95	86	76	70
10	20	62	55	47	42	16	19	101	92	82	74
						16	20	107	98	87	79
11	11	34	30	25	21						
11	12	38	33	28	24	17	17	96	87	77	70
11	13	42	37	31	27	17	18	102	92	82	75
11	14	46	40	34	30	17	19	109	99	88	81
11	15	50	44	37	33	17	20	115	105	93	86
11	16	54	47	41	36						
11	17	57	51	44	39	18	18	109	99	88	81
11	18	61	55	47	42	18	19	116	106	94	87
11	19	65	58	50	45	18	20	123	112	100	92
11	20	69	62	53	48						
						19	19	123	113	101	93
						19	20	130	119	107	99
						20	20	138	127	114	105

RANDOM SAMPLING NUMBERS

	1	2	3	4	5	6	7	8	9	10	11	12	13	14	15	16
1	0	6	2	8	3	5	7	6	4	9	0	7	6	6	8	0
2	3	4	2	5	2	0	3	0	5	1	5	1	3	5	7	1
3	3	4	7	4	1	5	8	8	9	9	4	0	3	6	3	6
4	4	7	5	0	4	8	3	3	0	5	7	4	8	4	5	9
5	9	3	5	6	8	1	1	7	2	0	7	8	3	5	8	6
6	8	6	1	5	7	5	3	7	6	6	4	9	5	0	7	1
7	2	0	2	3	0	7	1	2	1	4	3	6	2	6	5	0
8	0	3	3	4	7	5	8	2	0	0	8	7	4	4	1	8
9	2	0	4	2	6	0	5	7	9	4	8	5	4	6	0	3
10	6	5	3	3	1	1	0	3	6	9	0	2	7	3	1	7
11	3	9	2	9	8	9	5	4	4	6	4	6	8	6	3	3
12	7	2	2	1	8	4	5	9	5	6	5	9	2	5	3	2
13	7	4	0	7	3	7	4	0	6	8	6	5	8	1	8	9
14	9	1	2	2	8	0	3	9	9	8	1	5	7	4	7	9
15	1	9	9	8	9	3	9	4	4	2	2	1	4	6	5	7
16	7	2	9	4	6	1	6	7	9	8	7	5	3	7	4	6
17	9	1	5	2	3	0	2	6	5	8	1	2	2	3	7	9
18	6	9	3	4	5	2	8	0	9	2	4	7	9	2	9	6
19	6	2	1	6	5	6	2	9	5	3	2	7	4	1	0	8
20	0	7	4	1	1	6	0	6	2	1	8	2	7	8	3	7

TABLE OF 't'

Degrees of freedom	SIGNIFICANCE LEVELS			
	0.10 (0.05, 1 tail)	0.05 (2 tails)	0.02 (0.01, 1 tail)	0.01 (2 tails)
1	6.314	12.706	31.821	63.657
2	2.920	4.303	6.965	9.925
3	2.353	3.182	4.541	5.841
4	2.132	2.776	3.747	4.604
5	2.015	2.571	3.365	4.032
6	1.943	2.447	3.143	3.707
7	1.895	2.365	2.998	3.499
8	1.860	2.306	2.896	3.355
9	1.833	2.262	2.821	3.250
10	1.812	2.228	2.764	3.169
11	1.796	2.201	2.718	3.106
12	1.782	2.179	2.681	3.055
13	1.771	2.160	2.650	3.012
14	1.761	2.145	2.624	2.977
15	1.753	2.131	2.602	2.947
16	1.746	2.120	2.583	2.921
17	1.740	2.110	2.567	2.898
18	1.734	2.101	2.552	2.878
19	1.729	2.093	2.539	2.861
20	1.725	2.086	2.528	2.845
21	1.721	2.080	2.518	2.831
22	1.717	2.074	2.508	1.819
23	1.714	2.069	2.500	2.807
24	1.711	2.064	2.492	2.797
25	1.708	2.060	2.485	2.787
26	1.706	2.056	2.479	2.779
27	1.703	2.052	2.473	2.771
28	1.701	2.048	2.467	2.763
29 or more (equivalent to z)	1.600	2.000	2.300	2.600

THE χ^2 DISTRIBUTION

Degrees of freedom	SIGNIFICANCE LEVELS					
	0.99	0.95	0.10 (0.05 in 1 tail)	0.05 (in 1 tail)	0.02 (0.01 in 1 tail)	0.01 (in 1 tail)
1	.00157	.00393	2.706	3.841	5.412	6.635
2	.0201	.103	4.605	5.991	7.824	9.210
3	.115	.352	6.251	7.815	9.837	11.340
4	.297	.711	7.779	9.488	11.668	13.277
5	.554	1.145	9.236	11.070	13.388	15.086
6	.872	1.635	10.645	12.592	15.033	16.812
7	1.239	2.167	12.017	14.067	16.622	18.475
8	1.646	2.733	13.362	15.507	18.168	20.090
9	2.088	3.325	14.684	16.919	19.679	21.666
10	2.558	3.940	15.987	18.307	21.161	23.209
11	3.053	4.575	17.275	19.675	22.618	24.725
12	3.571	5.226	18.549	21.026	24.054	26.217
13	4.107	5.892	19.812	22.362	25.472	27.688
14	4.660	6.571	21.064	23.685	26.873	29.141
15	5.229	7.261	22.307	24.996	28.259	30.578
16	5.812	7.962	23.542	26.296	29.633	32.000
17	6.408	8.672	24.769	27.587	30.995	33.409
18	7.015	9.390	25.989	28.869	32.346	34.805
19	7.633	10.117	27.204	30.144	33.687	36.191
20	8.260	10.851	28.412	31.410	35.020	37.566